Preventing Misdiagnosis of Women

Women's Mental Health and Development

Series Editor: Barbara F. Okun, *Northeastern University*

Women's Mental Health and Development covers therapeutic issues of current relevance to women. This book series offers up-to-date, practical, culture-sensitive, professional resources for counseolors, social workers, psychologists, nurse practitioners, family therapists, and others in the helping professions. Volumes in this series are also of significant value to scholars in gender studies and women's studies.

This series is designed to deal particularly with those issues and populations underrepresented in the current professional literature. Particular attention is paid to the sociocultural contexts of these issues and populations. While some of the volumes of this series cover topics pertinent to all women, others focus on topics applicable to specific groups. The series integrates material from established models, emerging theoretical constructs, and solid empirical findings in a format designed to be applicable for clinical practice. Professionals and trainees in a variety of mental health fields will find these readable, user-friendly volumes immediately useful.

Authors of volumes in this series are selected on the basis of their scholarship and clinical expertise. The editorial board is composed of leading clinicians and scholars from psychology, counseling, and social work.

Editorial Board

Preventing Misdiagnosis of Women

A Guide to Physical Disorders That Have Psychiatric Symptoms

Elizabeth A. Klonoff
Hope Landrine

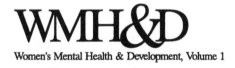

Women's Mental Health & Development, Volume 1

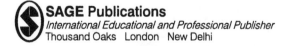

SAGE Publications
International Educational and Professional Publisher
Thousand Oaks   London   New Delhi

For information address:

 SAGE Publications, Inc.
2455 Teller Road
Thousand Oaks, California 91320
E-mail: order@sagepub.com

SAGE Publications Ltd.
6 Bonhill Street
London EC2A 4PU
United Kingdom

SAGE Publications India Pvt. Ltd.
M-32 Market
Greater Kailash I
New Delhi 110 048 India

Printed in the United States of America

Library of Congress Cataloging-in-Publication Data

Klonoff, Elizabeth A.
    Preventing misdiagnosis of women: A guide to physical
disorders that have psychiatric symptoms / Elizabeth
A. Klonoff, Hope Landrine.
        p.   cm.—(Women's mental health and development; vol. 1)
    Includes bibliographical references and index.
    ISBN 0-7619-0046-2 (cloth: alk. paper).—ISBN 0-7619-0047-0
(pbk.: alk. paper)
    1. Psychological manifestations of general diseases. 2. Women—
Mental health. 3. Mental illness—Physiological aspects.
4. Psychiatric errors. 5. Diagnostic errors. I. Landrine, Hope,
1954- . II. Title. III. Series.
RC455.4.B5K56 1996
616.89'0082—dc20   96-25183

This book is printed on acid-free paper.

    98 99 00 01 02 10 9 8 7 6 5 4 3 2

Acquiring Editor: Jim Nageotte
Editorial Assistant: Nancy Hale
Production Editor: Sherrise M. Purdum
Typesetter & Designer: Andrea D. Swanson
Indexer: Teri Greenberg
Cover Designer: Ravi Balasuriya

This book is dedicated to our teachers whose lessons made it possible: To Muriel Lezak for introducing me to the importance of physical and neuro-psychological disorders, modeling how to talk to and acquire the cooperation of physicians, and showing me how to introduce psychological issues to patients with serious medical conditions; Anthony Biglan for teaching me to always question the true cause of everything; and Murray Sidman for proving to me that being scientific and data based is the operational definition of caring.

—*Elizabeth A. Klonoff*

To Al Berman for teaching me about neuropsychology and physical disorders and making me forever question functional etiologies; (the late) Stanley Milgram for teaching me attribution theory; Bill Hancur for introduc-ing me to temporal lobe epilepsy; Phil Zimbardo for teaching me about the role of causal attributions in psychiatric symptoms; and Bernice Lott for teaching me more than I possibly could list.

—*Hope Landrine*

Contents

PART II: Seizure Disorders

PART III: Other Disorders

PART IV: Clinical Practice Considerations

Acknowledgments

We express grateful acknowledgment of the publishers below for their permission to reprint figures and illustrations from the following:

Table 4.1 is from "Clinical and Electroencephological Classification of Epileptic Seizures," by H. Gasaut, 1970, *Epilepsia, 1,* p. 102. Adapted with permission of the publisher.

Figure 5.1 is from *Dynamic Anatomy and Physiology* (4th ed.), by L. L. Langley, J. R. Telford, and J. B. Christensen, 1974, p. 229, St. Louis: Mosby Year Book, Inc. Reprinted with permission of the publisher.

Figure 5.2 is from *The Human Nervous System: Introduction and Review* (4th ed.), by C. R. Noback, N. L. Strominger, and R. J. Demarest, 1991, Philadelphia: Lea & Febiger. Reprinted with permission of first and third authors and publisher.

Figure 8.1 is from *Functional Human Anatomy* (2nd ed.), by J. E. Crouch, 1972, p. 480, Philadelphia: Lea & Febiger. Reprinted with permission of the publisher.

Figure 8.2 is from *Pathophysiology: Clinical Concepts of Disease Processes* (4th ed.), by S. A. Price and L. M. Wilson, 1992, p. 374, St. Louis: Mosby Year Book, Inc. Reprinted with permission of the publisher.

Introduction: A Case of Borderline Personality Disorder?

One of the first cases that I (Hope Landrine) saw, as a new, young clinician still practicing under supervision, was a 27-year-old, single, White woman who had a long history of psychiatric difficulties. Kate had seen six local therapists (of various theoretical orientations, feminist therapists included) over the past 3 years and despised them, she said, because they were stupid and incompetent—they didn't help her get better. She hoped I'd do a better job and, indeed, she felt sure that I would. These statements, my young clinical insight told me, were a sign that Kate probably had a borderline personality disorder, a disorder entailing (among other things) the tendency to quickly devalue and despise or, alternatively, to idealize others (e.g., her prior therapists and myself, respectively)—a set of problems in relating to others that is difficult to change.

After assessment and interview, it seemed that Kate *was* suffering from a borderline personality disorder: She had a long history of intense and unstable relationships in which she'd fallen in love instantly with someone she immediately idealized and then within a matter of days, weeks, or months came to thoroughly despise. She flew into a rage when these lovers failed to meet her unrealistic expectations of them and then threatened them, abused them verbally and physically, threw them out of her apartment, and finally sank into an intense, suicidal depression that never lasted long. She could not tolerate being without a companion or lover for long and became suicidal and depressed without one, yet always seemed to find another quickly. Consequently, she was either intensely happy and "in love"; bitter, angry, and in a rage; or depressed—each equally frequently. She was uncertain about nearly everything in her life, including what she wanted to do or be and her sexual orientation. She was a perpetual student who had been in college for 9 years but had yet to obtain a bachelor's degree because she changed her college major about once per semester; she changed her sexual partners with equal frequency. She engaged in numerous, potentially self-damaging acts, such as driving drunk, getting into fistfights and brawls, and some self-mutilation, including burning herself with cigarettes and making (purposefully nonlethal but bloody and ugly) scars on herself with a razor blade. Her sexual behavior consisted largely of hit-and-run sex with strangers and included men, women, groups, objects, and some sadomasochistic acts. All of the latter she said she did in a desperate attempt to *feel* something sexual: She had almost no genital sensations and had never experienced sexual pleasure or orgasm with women or men. She had recently decided to relinquish these sexual acts because she'd always seen them as morally wrong. She entertained the idea that perhaps one wasn't *supposed* to feel sexual pleasure because it was sinful. Perhaps her virtual absence of genital sensations was verification of her underlying belief that she was morally superior to others; perhaps she'd give up sex altogether.

Thus, unlike most borderline personalities whose uncertainty about themselves includes uncertainty about their values, Kate was very clear about her values, about her sense of right and wrong. Indeed, it is accurate to say that she was moralistic: She weighed everything, no matter how inconsequential, in terms of its goodness or rightness; elevated the trivial to the status of a moral issue; and immediately categorized people along moral lines as all good or all bad (only to later suddenly shift them from one of these categories to the other). Consequently, whenever she tried to make a decision about anything (e.g., whether to read a particular book, whether to tell her boss what she thought of him), the issue inevitably became one of right versus wrong, good versus bad. This rendered decision making difficult at best and led to incessant ruminating about the moral correctness of *all* of her current and past decisions: She could not decide if something she'd recently done or said was good or bad, if her parents were good or bad, if her current lover was good or bad, if her thoughts about some person meant that she herself was good or bad, if her instructor was good or bad (etc.), and she wrote all of these thoughts and moral ruminations down in enormous detail in a huge collection of journals that were numbered consecutively and carefully catalogued.

On the Minnesota Multiphasic Personality Inventory (MMPI), she scored 2-4-7-8 (with Scales 2 and 4 in the low 70s and Scales 7 and 8 in the mid 60s), a profile that purportedly is common in those suffering from borderline personality disorder.[1] On the Rorschach (scored by Exner criteria), all of her responses included Form, but there were many Color-Dominated Form responses (with poor Form) and a statistically greater than normal number of Achromatic Color responses—all, again, consistent with borderline personality disorder. True, she had a few obsessive symptoms (the moralistic ruminating, the keeping of voluminous notebooks, the indecisiveness), but these nonetheless fell far short of the criteria for an obsessive disorder of any type and so were dismissed as relatively unimportant. We conceptualized Kate as a woman suffering from borderline personality disorder—as a very troubled woman whose major problematic behaviors included (but were not limited to) inability to make decisions, episodic depression, episodic rage and dyscontrol, incessant ruminating, poor social skills (all of which affected her ability to hold a job), inability to maintain a relationship with anyone, and a sexual dysfunction.

Thus, we developed a careful, eclectic treatment plan to address these multiple problems. The treatment included some insight-oriented therapy as well as cognitive-behavioral and behavioral interventions. We also suggested that she see someone who specialized in sex therapy for assessment of the cause of and treatment of her sexual dysfunction, and we gave her a referral. We discussed family therapy, but she had no interest in it. In short, a variety of interventions were used. She participated actively and cooperatively in her therapy, without resistance, attempts to sabotage it, or any efforts to manipulate me. She was very interested in the therapy, in fact, and asked for books she could read about the various behavioral interventions in particular, books from which she took copious notes (which she brought to her sessions) and about which she then asked an enormous number of questions. She came to all of her sessions on time, never missed a session, did all of her therapeutic homework, and worked very hard in therapy. In light of the range of interventions employed and her genuine, sincere, and active commitment to changing her behavior, she should have gotten better. She didn't.

Kate not only showed no improvement in 4 months of weekly therapy (in the 12 to 16 sessions in which some improvement, according to psychotherapy outcome data, should have been seen), she got progressively worse. Her depressions became longer, more frequent, more severe, and unrelated to the loss of a lover. She began to complain of feeling that there was something wrong with her memory and perhaps her mind in general. She was more disheveled and seemed increasingly "out of it" (for lack of a better description), and her speech became increasingly tangential and circumstantial as well—or perhaps I simply started to notice it. My supervisors and I were concerned that her depression was becoming deeper and potentially dangerous, so we considered prescribing antidepressant medication, which would be suggested to her at her next session.

Simultaneously, as Kate became worse, I became increasingly concerned about her and began to seriously doubt the efficacy of the treatments—after all, she was getting worse despite the various therapies. Why wasn't she getting any better? Would a more strictly behavioral approach be more successful? What was I missing? I raised these questions with my clinical supervisors and their collective response was that I was expecting too much change too soon. Personality disorders, they said, are lifelong, maladaptive, and self-limiting ways of behaving and as such, by definition, don't change overnight. Her depression, in this context (related to her behavior rather than to losing a lover), may not be as bad a sign as it appears: It could be a sign of improvement, of self-evaluation and insight, or even of "regression in service of the ego." If she truly were deteriorating, my supervisors said, some kind of psychosis would have appeared by now; it hadn't.

An Alternative Conceptualization (Diagnosis)

Unsatisfied with those responses, I complained about all of this to a professor and friend, a clinical psychologist and neuropsychologist. I explained Kate's symptoms and problems, my interventions, how she was getting worse instead of better, and how I felt increasingly baffled by all of it. He quietly reminded me that I was doing all of the best interventions and seemed to be doing everything that could be done. I pressed him, "If I'm doing all the best interventions for this problem, then *why* is she getting worse?" His response was,

> Perhaps you're doing all the right interventions but for the wrong problem, for a problem that this woman does not have. If you do everything right to change a problem but it doesn't change at all, then you have the wrong problem in mind, and so the therapy is useless. She probably isn't a borderline personality at all, and that's why she isn't getting better. Your diagnosis, your conceptualization of what's going on with her is wrong.

That was a surprise to me. I pressed for more.

He then suggested that Kate probably had some symptoms that were inconsistent with the diagnosis of borderline personality disorder and with my conceptualization of her problems but that I'd decided to ignore those symptoms (not in terms of treating them—for each symptom was treated—but in my theoretical understanding of her difficulties). That was true: In addition to being obsessively moralistic and exhibiting some obsessive behaviors, she lacked genital sensations even when nondepressed and masturbating; that was something I'd never seen before, and it didn't make any more sense to me than it did to the sex therapist whom Kate was seeing conjointly. I told him this. His response was to explain that there were several neurological, endocrinological, and other physical disorders that manifested themselves in psychiatric symptoms—and in her symptoms in particular. He suggested that she had temporal lobe epilepsy, a disorder that I'd never heard of and consequently knew nothing about. He described how this form of epilepsy entailed psychiatric symptoms instead of convulsions and how these psychiatric symptoms were, in some respects, analogous to a convulsion. Temporal lobe epilepsy could present in symptoms of personality disorder or depression or schizophrenia and could cause hallucinations and delusions and even lost time. He thought that her moralistic ruminating and obsessive writing of notes and journals did not reflect obsessive tendencies but instead were manifestations of the hyperethicality and hypergraphia[2] that were prototypical symptoms of temporal lobe epilepsy. He said that this type of epilepsy probably was extremely common in the general population because the temporal lobes were very sensitive and readily injured by anoxia at birth, delivery using forceps, or simply by having prolonged, high fevers as an infant. He suggested that I check Kate's early life history for such problems and find out what her birth weight had been; he assured me that I'd find evidence of early brain or central nervous system (CNS) injury or dysfunction. Given how easy it is to injure the temporal lobes, he suspected that up to half the population of the nation had undiagnosed temporal lobe epilepsy—or temporal lobe epilepsy that had been misdiagnosed as a psychiatric disorder. He promised me some materials on the topic the next day and suggested that I talk with my supervisors about having Kate sent for an electroencephalogram (EEG) instead of for a consultation for an antidepressant; an antidepressant would only make her symptoms worse if those symptoms were the result of an underlying, undiagnosed neurological disorder.

The following day, my neuropsychologist friend gave me a tattered out-of-print book to read (a book he'd read years ago as a graduate student), *Ictal and Subictal Neurosis: Diagnosis and Treatment* by A. D. Jonas (1965), along with copies of a few recent articles by David Bear and his colleagues (Bear, 1979a, 1979b; Bear & Fedio, 1977) and a little book by two neurologists, Benson and Blumer (1975). I read them quickly. To my surprise, Kate's symptoms were described in these materials in detail, with all of what I'd taken to be inconsistent symptoms included. Case study after case study.

Temporal lobe epilepsy. An epilepsy without convulsions, with psychiatric symptoms such as depression and classic "neurotic" disorders instead. I relayed all of this information to my supervisors who doubted its veracity and didn't like it at all. It was bunk, a bizarre idea, they said—how come *they'd* never heard of this disorder before, they asked. In the end however, they accepted temporal lobe epilepsy as a possibility solely because, they said, the neuropsychologist was a respected colleague of theirs; had he not been, this new conceptualization would have been rejected. After considerable discussion, my supervisors agreed that I could explain all of this to Kate and suggest that she have an EEG—if and only if her early history revealed evidence of the brain injury that the neuropsychologist was sure would be found.

In my next session with Kate, I asked her about her birth and infancy, unusual questions that therapists are not ordinarily trained to ask and that neither I nor my clinical supervisors had ever asked of a person being seen in therapy. To my surprise, Kate revealed that she had been a low-birth-weight, premature infant of a twin birth (her sister died 2 days after their birth), born to a mother who had pneumonia at the time of delivery. Kate had been maintained in an incubator for a period (she was not sure of how long but volunteered to find out from her mother) and was critically ill with her mother's infection during the first month or so of her life, with prolonged high fevers and infantile seizures. After acquiring this information, I explained the possibility of temporal lobe epilepsy to Kate. She was extraordinarily pleased by the idea, delighted in fact with the possibility of having a neurological disorder, and happy to have an EEG, something she wanted as soon as possible. She said she hoped that the EEG would be positive and that she would be discovered to have this strange type of epilepsy. In part, this was because she wanted there to be a simple cause and solution to her problems, as anyone does. Mostly, however, she hoped her EEG would be positive because she wanted her problem to be neurological rather than psychiatric. The former is a far less stigmatizing category, casting little shame on her or on her family. This response is one that both authors have seen nearly 100% of the time, especially among the parents of disturbed children and adolescents.

One week later, Kate had an EEG that was positive for abnormal discharges in the temporal lobes, bilaterally—temporal lobe epilepsy. We referred Kate to a local neurologist for adjunctive treatment. She was placed on Tegretol as well as on an additional anticonvulsant (seizure medication). Within 4 weeks, she was, in many respects, a different person; I felt as if I were sitting with someone I'd never met before. She was changed and was free of her most bizarre symptoms, the depression and rage foremost among those. Certainly, she still had several interpersonal and other difficulties that required therapy. She had, after all, gone through her life with a neurological disorder that had altered the direction and nature of her behavior and of her development. Her interpersonal behavior, responses, and skills were consequently poor, and she had much to learn about interacting normally with others. Importantly, she had spent many years attributing her symptoms to her relationship with her parents (with the eager assistance and encouragement of therapists) and now needed to reattribute those symptoms to understand them in their neurological context. Her absence of genital sensations, her sudden depressions and rages all needed to be thought through and worked through again. After all, she had come up with *reasons* for being depressed, things in her life that she believed to be causes of her depression. Now, these had to be thought through again and new attributions made because none of these things was the cause—the cause was neurological.[3] She had, in effect, a plethora of residual and reactive symptoms that needed therapeutic attention. But her major problem and the etiology of her problems, a seizure disorder, were under control.

Fortunately for Kate, I had a friend who led me to the right diagnosis and to the proper treatment, who led me to reconceptualize the source of her problems as physical rather than psychiatric or social. Without him, Kate may have continued for the rest of her life in treatment with countless therapists, making no progress whatsoever and with that lack of progress blamed on her, until she deteriorated enough to hallucinate and be confined to a psychiatric hospital as incurable and severely disabled, where she would no doubt remain. Preventing this kind of misdiagnosis—this misattribution of symptoms to psychiatric rather than to physical causes—is important for the welfare of women in therapy and of therapists alike and has obvious relevance to rising health care costs. Preventing this kind of misdiagnosis is what this book is about.

Purpose of This Book and Scope of the Problem

The purpose of this book is to provide therapists with information on physical disorders that are common but that present themselves in psychiatric symptoms. By "physical disorders" we mean underlying, undeniable, serious, pathological physical processes, such as temporal lobe epilepsy, multiple sclerosis, or disorders of the thyroid gland; we mean physical disorders that are well-known in medicine and so have medical names, physical etiologies, and (often) simple cures; we mean physical disorders that—if not diagnosed and treated properly—can result in a woman's being confined to a mental hospital for her entire life or even result in her untimely death. The major symptoms of these purely physical disorders are psychiatric, however. The major symptoms are chronic depression, anxiety, or both; anorexia, periods of lost time, emotional lability, panic attacks, and a host of other complaints that women (far more often than men) present to their therapists. *Because* the symptoms of these physical disorders are psychiatric and emotional rather than physical, women tend to seek assistance and help from therapists rather than from physicians. As Kate did, most women assume that depression or anxiety is necessarily a sign of a psychological or psychosocial disturbance and never entertain the possibility that these instead may be symptoms of a purely physical disturbance. Unfortunately, their therapists tend to make the same assumption: Often, therapists do not entertain the idea that the root of a woman's anxiety or depression could be an endocrinological disorder (for example) that has yet to be diagnosed and treated, and the consequences of that error range from serious to lethal. Our purpose in this book is to inform therapists about these physical disorders and to encourage them to consider these as possible causes of the symptoms and complaints of the women they see in therapy. Our goal is to prevent the misdiagnosis (the erroneous conceptualization) of these physical disorders as psychiatric, to prevent women from sitting in therapy for problems that cannot possibly be alleviated by that therapy no matter the type, and to improve and save women's lives by so doing.

By the term *misdiagnosis* we do not mean the use of the wrong psychiatric label for a problem that is more accurately described by a different label from the *Diagnostic and Statistical Manual of Mental Disorders (DSM)*. Rather, by misdiagnosis, we mean the initial classifying of a woman's symptoms and their cause as psychiatric[4] (and therefore amenable to counseling or psychotherapy) rather than as purely physical and in need of medical attention. This classifying of a woman's symptoms and their causes as psychiatric rather than physical is the most basic decision that every therapist makes; because this initial classification determines whether therapy (treatment) is conducted or not, *it is a diagnosis* even though no *DSM* labels are involved. This diagnosing of a woman's symptoms and their causes as psychiatric necessarily is rendered by *every therapist about every woman being seen in therapy* and is the explanation, the reason for seeing that woman in therapy—even though the therapist may reject diagnostic labels on political or scientific grounds. Yet this fundamental diagnosis without *DSM* labels can be wrong, it can be a misdiagnosis because the problem may be physical, as in Kate's case.

The Frequency of Misdiagnosis

There are ample reasons to suspect that the misdiagnosis of a physical disorder as psychiatric is rampant, for women in therapy in particular. Indeed, we suspect that such misdiagnoses account for the hundreds of thousands of children and adults who are relegated to back wards of mental hospitals and other institutions for those with chronic disorders; for the millions of ostensibly incurable outpatients of community mental health centers across the nation; and for the millions of bizarre, disturbed, homeless, ostensibly "mentally ill" of the nation's cities. Evidence regarding how rampant this kind of misdiagnosis is comes from a few reliable sources. One example is an article by Hoffman (1982) in the *Journal of the American Medical Association,* who reported on 215 consecutive new admissions to a psychiatric hospital in San Francisco. All 215 patients were given psychiatric diagnoses and treated for psychiatric disorders, with medication often included. Later neurologic examinations of these patients found that *41%* of them had neurological and other physical disorders that no one had checked for and that subsequently were misdiagnosed as psychiatric. These misdiagnoses were clinically significant insofar as they led not only to useless treatment (to therapy and drug treatments that could not alter the underlying physical cause of the symptoms) but to treatment that exacerbated the physical disorder and so was harmful to the patient.

Likewise, Weinberger, Wagner, and Wyatt (1983), in a well-known, comprehensive review article in *Schizophrenia Bulletin* concluded that up to 83% of people diagnosed as schizophrenic instead have lesions (tumors) or seizures in the temporal lobes; computerized tomography (CT) scan and postmortem analyses of their brains have typically found such temporal lobe pathology. Blumer (1970) and Hall, Popkin, Devaul, Faillace, and Stickney (1978) similarly discussed the variety of common physical disorders that are frequently misdiagnosed as psychiatric. Finally, in an address delivered at the annual convention of the American Psychological Association a few years ago (summarized in the *APA Monitor*), Joan Rittenhouse of the National Institute of Mental Health concluded from such studies that up to 81% of all psychiatric patients (inpatients and outpatients) probably have misdiagnosed physical disorders, with misdiagnosed cancers a frequent and lethal diagnostic error. She indicated that lawsuits were increasing against therapists for failing to investigate a possible physical disorder among patients that they had been seeing for more than a year.

These studies estimate that 41% to 83% of people being treated for psychiatric disorders have misdiagnosed physical disorders. The prevalence of such misdiagnoses may be higher or lower than these studies indicate; may vary with the social class, age, and ethnicity of the woman seeking treatment; and may even vary with the training and the theoretical orientation of the therapist. We do not know if any or all of these factors are involved in light of the nature and dearth of studies on such misdiagnoses; the few existing studies of misdiagnosis did not investigate the role of social class, ethnicity, gender, and other variables. Yet, again, we can say from these studies that 41% to 83% of people being treated for psychiatric disorders instead may have misdiagnosed physical disorders and that such figures are frightening whether they vary with status or not. The purpose of this book is to address this widespread problem.

Why the Focus on Women?

Because women frequent therapists far more often than do men (Russo, 1995), the misdiagnosis of physical disorders as psychiatric is a women's issue, and so this book focuses on women. That is not meant to suggest that men who have physical disorders are not misdiagnosed as having psychiatric ones too but, rather, that women are misdiagnosed in this manner significantly more often than men simply because the majority of people in therapy are women. In addition, the vast majority of the physical disorders that we describe here are manifested solely in symptoms of depression, anxiety, or somatization. These symptoms and disorders are significantly more common among women than among men (Russo, 1995), and this gender difference in the prevalence of these specific symptoms and disorders has yet to be sufficiently explained. Thus, we present the novel hypothesis that *the misdiagnosis of physical disorders as psychiatric in part accounts for women's higher rate of depression, anxiety, and somatization disorders,* as discussed below.

Explaining Women's Symptoms

It is well-known that women are significantly more likely than men to exhibit a variety of psychiatric symptoms, symptoms of depression and anxiety foremost among those (Landrine, 1992; McGrath, Strickland, Keita, & Russo, 1990; Rickel, Gerrad, & Iscoe, 1984). Indeed, depression is the single most common diagnosis received by women who seek mental health services, whether they are White, Black, or Latino, and anxiety and somatization symptoms are also frequent.[5] That women are more likely than men to exhibit these specific symptoms and disorders is undeniable, and so the question then becomes "Why?" *Why* do women exhibit significantly more frequent depressive, anxiety-related, and somatization symptoms and disorders than do men?

There are a variety of competing theories regarding women's higher rate of these specific symptoms and disorders,[6] as well as some reliable empirical evidence. That empirical evidence suggests two reasons that women exhibit these symptoms and disorders more frequently than do men. The first is that women's rate of exposure to generic (can happen to anyone) stressful life events and life crises is significantly higher than that of men, and such stressors (e.g., problems with children, responsibility for others, death of a loved one, poverty, unemployment, and underemployment, etc.) are known to contribute to depression, anxiety, and other symptoms for everyone—men, women, and children alike (see Lazarus, 1966; Lazarus & Launier, 1978; Thoits, 1984). Thus, women may have higher rates of these stress-related, psychiatric disorders simply because women experience significantly more stress than men do.[7] Although this gender difference in exposure to stressful life events and crises in part explains women's higher rate of stress-related (anxiety, depression) symptoms (Kessler, Price, & Wortman, 1985), it does not seem sufficient explanation for women's extraordinarily high rates of these disorders and symptoms, and thus additional explanations are needed (Klonoff & Landrine, 1995; Landrine, Klonoff, Gibbs, Manning, & Lund, 1995).

A second reason that women's rate of these stress-related symptoms and disorders far exceeds that of men is that, *in addition to* experiencing higher rates of generic stress, women also experience gender-specific stress—stressful life events that women experience but that men do not (Russo, 1995). Two general types of gender-specific stressors have been investigated and demonstrated to erode women's physical and mental health. The first are role-related stressors, such as the multiple-role strain, role overload, and role conflict that women—but not men—who are employed, married, and have children experience.[8] The second type are brutal and physical gender-specific stressors (Russo, 1995), including battering, rape, sexual harassment, and other forms of violence against women (Goodman, Koss, & Russo, 1993; Koss, Koss, & Woodruff, 1991). Studies suggest that including both of these gender-specific stressors along with the more generic ones increases our ability to predict and explain stress-related symptoms and disorders among women as well as women's higher rate of these symptoms. Researchers have been suggesting that attempts to understand stress-related symptoms among women that ignore the reality of ongoing (sexist) gender-specific stressors are as limited and inadequate as attempts to understand stress-related symptoms among Blacks while ignoring the meaning of race and the prevalence of racism (Landrine, Klonoff, Gibbs, Manning, & Lund, 1995; Russo, 1995).

The aforementioned research provides two variables that might explain why women exhibit depression, anxiety, and somatization disorders far more often than men do. Our own recent studies suggest a third reason—namely, women also experience subtle sexist discrimination (e.g., being called "a bitch," being treated as if they're stupid, being told sexist jokes) that men do not, and this is an additional source of gender-specific stress that contributes to women's symptoms (Klonoff & Landrine, 1995). Recent studies using our measure of such sexist discrimination (the *Schedule of Sexist Events,* Klonoff & Landrine, 1995) revealed, for example, that such subtle sexism accounts for more of the variance in women's symptoms than do the generic stressors that are known to be powerful predictors of women's symptoms. Specifically, we found that subtle sexist acts were the best predictor of symptoms of anxiety, depression, and somatization among our culturally diverse sample of 631 women (Landrine et al., 1995). However, even when we added generic stressors to sexist acts (sexist events), we at best could account for 50% of the variance in women's symptoms (correlations of $R = .70$ to .73). Although this is considerable, our findings nonetheless mean that something else is going on, that there are additional variables (yet to be addressed) that predict and explain (the remaining 50% of the variance in) women's significantly higher rate of depression, anxiety, and somatization.

Thus, in this book, we suggest another potentially powerful variable that may help explain why women's rate of depression, anxiety, and somatization far exceeds that of men: This variable is the physical disorders (many of which are more common among women than men) that manifest themselves in such symptoms but are misdiagnosed and treated as psychiatric 41% to 83% of the time simply because therapists are not aware of them and are not screening for them.

Disorders of Focus

In this book, we focus on two types of physical disorders. The first are purely physical disorders that are known to be highly frequent among women, known to be significantly more frequent among women than among men, and known to present in psychiatric symptoms, of depression and anxiety in particular. These physical disorders are the most important to consider because they obviously have the highest probability of being misdiagnosed as psychiatric and no doubt play a role in women's higher rate of (ostensible) psychiatric disorders. The second type are physical disorders that are *not known* to be more frequent among women than among men but nonetheless present in the symptoms that women exhibit far more often than do men (depression, anxiety, anorexia). These disorders also have a high probability of being misdiagnosed as psychiatric (but perhaps a lower probability than that of the former disorders) and may account for an additional, small percentage of the variance in gender differences in rates of depression, anxiety, and similar disorders.

Source of Data

For the past 15 years, we have investigated literature on physical disorders of every type, searching for those that might have psychiatric symptoms. To our surprise and dismay, there are many disorders like this, physical disorders with names and with specific physical treatments—cures. But this information remains buried, hidden in articles and books that most therapists would never read: textbooks of neurology, internal medicine, and endocrinology, and journals such as *Epilepsia* and *Archives of Neurology and Psychiatry.* In the pages that follow, we summarize the information that we have gathered from these medical journals and textbooks. We describe and explain the most common physical disorders that present in psychiatric-behavioral symptoms and complaints of depression, anxiety, somatization, anorexia, "hysteria," "histrionic personality," and "lost time" in particular—the symptoms most commonly presented by women. We detail the additional symptoms that the therapist should look for as well as specific questions that can be asked, to prevent misdiagnosis of these physical disorders as psychiatric. In some cases, we also detail the scores on psychological tests that will assist psychologists in differentiating physical from psychiatric disorder. Where appropriate, we discuss the psychiatric medications that will exacerbate and, indeed, *can cause and precipitate* these physical disorders, and we present cases from our previous experience in hospitals and clinics, our private practice, and the local news as illustrations of the patterns of symptoms seen.

The chapters here are organized by major types of physical disorders. The disorders that we cover are not the only physical disorders that present as psychiatric; there are several others. We have selected those that, in our collective clinical experience and according to the epidemiological data, are most common in the population. The information presented in each chapter is summarized from hundreds of medical sources. To facilitate reading the chapters, we have not cited these innumerable references throughout the text. Rather, a few references are cited and appear at the end of each chapter; then the entire set of references used to write the chapters is provided in the bibliography. Where appropriate, we have also provided some references in endnotes, as we've done in this Introduction. Each chapter is written in practical, nontechnical language. Any technical terminology, as well as anatomy and physiology, are explained in each chapter and defined in the Glossary at the end of this book. The reader will need to know and must learn to use these terms to communicate with and understand the communications of medical practitioners.

In addition, Chapter 10 discusses how to interact with the internists, endocrinologists, neurologists, and other medical specialists whose cooperation is essential to acquiring a variety of tests and adjunctive treatment for women. The appendix summarizes the questions to ask women in order to rule out these physical disorders. It also includes a quick and practical symptom guide, with symptoms (e.g., depression, panic attacks) or psychiatric diagnoses (e.g., major affective disorder, bipolar disorder) as headers, and the physical disorders that present in that symptom listed beneath.

Finally, throughout this book, we refer to the people we have treated as "patients" for three reasons. The first is that we have both worked primarily in hospital settings where people in treatment tend to be called patients. The second is that, in our private practice, we have both referred countless people to physicians for what we suspected was actually a physical disorder—and the physicians always refer to them as patients. Thus, we refer to people as patients out of habit; the use of the word *patient* is not meant to imply allegiance to the medical model, for we both staunchly reject disease conceptualizations of problematic behavior. The third reason that we refer to people as patients throughout this book is that the endocrinologists, neurologists, and other medical specialists with whom the reader will need to interact in order to rule out the physical disorders presented here will invariably refer to people as patients and expect the reader (when making a referral) to do so. It is to the reader's benefit to put aside any personal and political objections to the term *patient* (no matter how justified those objections are) and become accustomed to hearing and to using that term to facilitate cooperation from the medical specialists who are essential to acquiring the best treatment for women whom the reader sees in therapy. Likewise, the use of the term *misdiagnosis* throughout this book, like the use of the specific psychiatric labels (e.g., hysteria, bipolar disorder) that women with physical disorders may have had attributed to them erroneously, is meant as a realistic description of what is happening out there in the world to women, not as a reflection of our views on labels. Whether one immediately rejects psychiatric labels on political or empirical grounds will not alter the undeniable fact that hundreds of thousands of women receive these psychiatric labels every day and is irrelevant to our point—namely, that these labels are errors because the problem may be a physical one.

Last, we focus here solely on physical disorders that can be, and that we suspect are being, misdiagnosed as psychiatric and do not discuss the various types of sexism in women's lives as one of many causes of women's symptoms. Doing so does not mean that we view these physical disorders as playing a greater role in women's symptoms than sexism, for our own ongoing research highlights the importance of sexism. Rather, we focus on these physical disorders because they have been neglected by therapists for far too long as one of many possible hypotheses, and such neglect has been to the detriment of women, their families and loved ones, and their therapists alike.

Notes

1. Psychological test scores are provided throughout this book for the psychologists among the readers. A discussion of the reliability, validity, and meaning of these tests and scores on them will not be provided.

2. Hyperethicality means excess moralism, hypergraphia means excess writing; these and all other technical terms are defined in the Glossary of Technical Terms.

3. People always have explanations for their symptoms of anxiety or depression, and although reasonable, these in fact may not be the cause of their symptoms—which instead could be physical in origin. When they feel depressed, people search for an explanation, for something that could cause it, and of course, they find something. Who couldn't? Who among us cannot think of at least one thing in our lives to be depressed about (whether we are or are not depressed)? Thus, when a woman says she's depressed and gives good interpersonal and social reasons for it, how does the therapist know that the reasons given are the cause?

4. We use the term *psychiatric* to mean social, political, interpersonal, familial, societal, intrapersonal (or some combination of these) in origin.

5. For data on this, see Russo and Sobel (1981); Russo, Amaro, and Winter (1987); Myers et al. (1984); Robins et al. (1984); and in particular, Russo and Green (1993) for a comprehensive review and discussion.

6. For discussions of these theories, see Nolen-Hoeksema (1990), Russo and Green (1993), McGrath et al. (1990), and Weissman and Merikangas (1986).

7. For examples of such studies, see Aneshensel, Frerichs, and Clark (1981); Belle (1990); Cleary and Mechanic (1983); Kessler and McLeod (1984); McGrath et al. (1990); and Newmann (1986, 1987).

8. See Aneshensel (1986); Baruch and Barnett (1986); Pugliesi (1988); Reifman, Biernat, and Lang (1991); Repetti, Matthews, and Waldron (1989); Verbrugge (1986); and Waldron and Jacobs (1989).

References

Aneshensel, C. S. (1986). Marital and employment role-strain, social support, and depression among adult women. In S. Hobfoll (Ed.), *Stress, social support, and women* (pp. 99-114). Washington, DC: Hemisphere.

Aneshensel, C. S., Frerichs, R. R., & Clark, V. A. (1981). Family roles and sex differences in depression. *Journal of Health and Social Behavior, 22,* 379-393.

Baruch, G. K., & Barnett, R. (1986). Role quality, multiple role involvement, and psychological well-being in midlife women. *Journal of Personality and Social Psychology, 51,* 578-585.

Bear, D. (1979a). Temporal lobe epilepsy: A syndrome of sensory-limbic hyperconnection. *Cortex, 15,* 357-384.

Bear, D. (1979b). The temporal lobes: An approach to the study of organic behavioral changes. In M. Gazzaniga (Ed.), *Handbook of behavioral neurobiology and neuropsychology.* New York: Plenum.

Bear, D., & Fedio, P. (1977). Quantitative analysis of interictal behavior in temporal lobe epilepsy. *Archives of Neurology, 34,* 454-467.

Belle, D. (1990). Poverty and women's mental health. *American Psychologist, 49,* 384-389.

Benson, D. F., & Blumer, D. (Eds.). (1975). *Psychiatric aspects of neurologic disease.* New York: Grune & Stratton.

Blumer, D. (1970). Neurological states masquerading as psychoses. *Maryland State Medical Journal, 19,* 55-60.

Cleary, P. D., & Mechanic, D. (1983). Sex differences in psychological distress among married people. *Journal of Health and Social Behavior, 24,* 111-121.

Goodman, L. A., Koss, M. P., & Russo, N. F. (1993). Violence against women: Physical and mental health effects: Part I. Research findings. *Applied & Preventive Psychology: Current Scientific Perspectives, 2,* 111-121.

Hall, R. C. W., Popkin, M. K., Devaul, R., Faillace, L. A., & Stickney, S. K. (1978). Physical illness presented as psychiatric disease. *Archives of General Psychiatry, 35*(11), 1315-1320.

Hoffman, R. S. (1982). Diagnostic errors in the evaluations of behavioral disorders. *JAMA, 248*(8), 964-967.

Jonas, A. D. (1965). *Ictal and subictal neurosis: Diagnosis and treatment.* Springfield, IL: Charles C Thomas.

Kessler, R. C., & McLeod, J. D. (1984). Sex differences in vulnerability to undesirable life events. *American Sociological Review, 49,* 620-631.

Kessler, R. C., Price, R. H., & Wortman, C. B. (1985). Social factors in psychopathology: Stress, social support, and coping processes. *Annual Review of Psychology, 36,* 531-572.

Klonoff, E. A., & Landrine, H. (1995). The Schedule of Sexist Events: A measure of recent and lifetime sexist discrimination in women's lives. *Psychology of Women Quarterly, 19*(4), 439-472.

Koss, M. P., Koss, P. G., & Woodruff, W. J. (1991). Deleterious effects of criminal victimization on women's health and medical utilization. *Archives of Internal Medicine, 151,* 342-357.

Landrine, H. (1992). *The politics of madness.* New York: Peter Lang.

Landrine, H., Klonoff, E. A., Gibbs, J., Manning, V., & Lund, M. (1995). Physical and psychiatric correlates of gender discrimination: An application of the Schedule of Sexist Events. *Psychology of Women Quarterly, 19*(4), 473-492.

Lazarus, R. S. (1966). *Psychological stress and the coping process.* New York: McGraw-Hill.

Lazarus, R. S., & Launier, R. (1978). Stress-related transactions between person and environment. In L. A. Pervin & M. Lewis (Eds.), *Perspectives in interactional psychology* (pp. 287-327). New York: Plenum.

McGrath, E., Strickland, B. R., Keita, G. P., & Russo, N. F. (1990). *Women and depression: Risk factors and treatment issues.* Washington, DC: American Psychological Association.

Myers, J. K., Weissman, M. M., Tischler, G. L., Holzer, C. E., Leaf, P. J., Orvaschel, H., Anthony, J. C., Boyd, J. H., Burke, J. D., Kramer, M., & Stoltzman, R. (1984). Six-month prevalence of psychiatric disorders in three communities. *Archives of General Psychiatry, 41,* 959-967.

Newmann, J. P. (1986). Gender, life strains, and depression. *Journal of Health and Social Behavior, 27,* 161-178.

Newmann, J. P. (1987). Gender differences in vulnerability to depression. *Social Service Review, 61,* 447-468.

Nolen-Hoeksema, S. (1990). *Sex differences in depression.* Stanford, CA: Stanford University Press.

Pugliesi, K. (1988). Employment characteristics, social support, and well-being of women. *Women and Health, 14,* 35-58.

Reifman, A., Biernat, M., & Lang, E. (1991). Stress, social support, and health in married professional women with small children. *Psychology of Women Quarterly, 15,* 431-445.

Repetti, R. L., Matthews, K. A., & Waldron, I. (1989). Employment and women's health. *American Psychologist, 44,* 1394-1401.

Rickel, A. U., Gerrad, M., & Iscoe, I. (1984). *Social and psychological problems of women.* Washington, DC: Hemisphere.

Robins, L. N., Helzer, J. E., Weissman, M. M., Orvaschel, H., Gruenberg, E., Burke, J. D., & Regier, D. A. (1984). Lifetime prevalence of specific psychiatric disorders in three sites. *Archives of General Psychiatry, 41,* 949-958.

Russo, N. F. (1995). Women's mental health: Research agenda for the twenty-first century. In B. Brown, B. Kramer, P. Reiker, & C. Willie (Eds.), *Mental health, racism, and sexism* (pp. 373-396). Pittsburgh: University of Pittsburgh Press.

Russo, N. F., Amaro, H., & Winter, M. (1987). The use of inpatient mental health services by Hispanic women. *Psychology of Women Quarterly, 11*(4), 427-442.

Russo, N. F., & Green, B. L. (1993). Women and mental health. In F. L. Denmark & M. A. Paludi (Eds.), *Psychology of women: A handbook of issues and theories* (pp. 379-436). Westport, CT: Greenwood.

Russo, N. F., & Sobel, S. B. (1981). Sex differences in the utilization of mental health facilities. *Professional Psychology, 12,* 7-19.

Thoits, P. A. (1984). Explaining distributions of psychological vulnerability: Lack of social support in the face of life stress. *Social Forces, 63,* 463-481.

Verbrugge, L. (1986). Role burdens and physical health of women and men. *Women and Health, 11,* 47-77.

Waldron, I., & Jacobs, J. A. (1989). Effects of multiple roles on women's health. *Women and Health, 15,* 3-19.

Weinberger, D. R., Wagner, R. L., & Wyatt, R. J. (1983). Neuropathological studies of schizophrenia: A selective review. *Schizophrenia Bulletin, 9,* 193-212.

Weissman, M. M., & Merikangas, K. R. (1986). The epidemiology of anxiety and panic disorders: An update. *Journal of Clinical Psychiatry, 47*(6, Suppl.), 11-17.

PART I

Endocrinological Disorders

The Endocrinological System

Several of the physical disorders that present in psychiatric symptoms are endocrinological disorders—disorders of the endocrine system. To facilitate an understanding of these disorders, in this chapter we describe how the endocrine system works and how it goes wrong.

The Endocrine System

The human body has two types of glands: (a) *endocrine or ductless glands,* which secrete chemicals called *hormones* directly into the blood stream, and (b) *exocrine or duct glands,* whose products pass through special ducts to the outer body and do not enter the blood stream (e.g., sweat and tear glands). The two parts of the brain that control the endocrine glands, along with the endocrine glands themselves (often called target glands), are collectively called the endocrine system.

The two parts of the brain included in the endocrine system are the hypothalamus and the pituitary gland. The hypothalamus is a group of small nuclei (nerve cell bodies inside the brain or spinal cord) in the brain. The various nuclei of the hypothalamus lie along the base of the brain, above the roof of your mouth, and are contiguous with the pituitary gland. The hypothalamus controls several vital bodily functions, including temperature, sleep cycle, and respiratory activity. The hypothalamus also controls the pituitary gland by stimulating it with chemicals that act as orders or commands to increase or decrease its activity. When the pituitary receives these chemical orders from the hypothalamus, it sends these orders along (in chemical form)

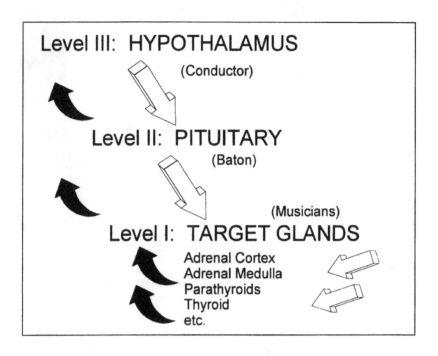

Figure 1.1. Feedback Loops in the Endocrinological System

to the target glands (e.g., the thyroid, the adrenals). The target glands respond to these chemical orders and messages from the pituitary by changing the output of their own chemicals. Such changes in the target glands are then communicated back to and read by the pituitary and the hypothalamus in a complex feedback system. The complexity of the feedback loops in the endocrine system is depicted in Figure 1.1.

These complex feedback loops might be best understood by thinking of the endocrine system as an orchestra. An orchestra has a conductor who is in charge and who determines how the music is played by the musicians. The musicians are seated in organized groups, such as the percussion section, the woodwinds, the horns, and the strings. The conductor determines how the music is played by pointing a baton at the various groups of musicians and directing them to play more slowly, loudly, or quickly. When the musicians follow those orders, the conductor stops pointing the baton at them; the conductor responds to their feedback. The endocrine system is quite similar. It has organized groups of musicians or glands (such as the adrenal, thyroid, pancreas, and parathyroid) that must work together in perfect harmony. It has a conductor, the hypothalamus, that determines how the music is played (which glands secrete, how much, and when). The hypothalamus controls these glands by pointing a baton, the pituitary gland, at the target glands. The target glands, like musicians, respond to the chemical orders of the baton and the conductor by changing their secretions (how loudly or quickly they play); this, in turn, alters the behavior of the conductor. When this communication system works well, the result is a beautifully complex, multidimensional physiological and psychological harmony. When it goes wrong, the outcome is physiological disharmony or noise—an endocrinological disorder.

When an orchestra plays horribly, the problem can be at any of several levels. The conductor might be drunk and, consequently, send the wrong messages to the right musicians; the baton could be warped and so send the right message to the wrong musicians; or any group or even several groups of the musicians could have problems following the music or the conductor. Disorders of the endocrine system are similar and can be the result of pathology (tumors, damage) at the level of the hypothalamus, pituitary, or in any of the target glands. If the problem in the endocrine system is at the level of the gland (Level I in Figure 1.1), the disorder is called a *primary* endocrinological disorder. If it is at the level of the pituitary (Level II), it is called a *secondary* endocrinological disorder, and if it is at the level of the hypothalamus (Level III), it is called a *tertiary* endocrinological disorder. Thus, for example, a patient might have primary, secondary, or tertiary hyperthyroidism.

The Endocrine Glands

Endocrine glands produce hormones, which are secreted directly into the blood. Thus, technically, hormones can be defined as the circulating chemical products of endocrine glands. Through circulation, hormones reach every tissue of the body. The types of endocrine glands relevant to this book are the pituitary, thyroid and parathyroid, pancreas, and adrenal glands. These particular glands appear in both sexes.

The pituitary gland is about the size of a peanut and is located at the base of the skull, suspended (hanging) from the hypothalamus. It has two sections that have very different functions. The posterior pituitary is directly behind a section of the optic (visual) nerve. A tumor in the posterior pituitary can result in visual defects or complete blindness. The posterior pituitary produces two hormones, antidiuretic hormone (ADH) and oxytocin. ADH regulates the kidneys' use of water. ADH also causes blood vessels to contract (close tightly and suddenly); this is called *vasoconstriction* of blood vessels. Thus, large amounts of ADH are often associated with hypertension. Oxytocin produces contractions of the uterus and facilitates lactation.

The anterior pituitary is thought to be controlled by hormones from the hypothalamus. It releases six of its own hormones: (a) adrenocorticotrophic hormone (ACTH), (b) human growth hormone, (c) thyrotropic hormone, (d) prolactin, and (e & f) two gonadotrophic hormones. These six hormones are not related to the disorders of focus and so will not be covered. Likewise, disorders of the pituitary (as the cause of endocrinological disorders) are somewhat rare, so the various functions of the pituitary will not be detailed here. The reader is referred to *Textbook of Endocrinology* by R. H. Williams (1981) for discussions of the pituitary. One pituitary disorder, however, hypopituitarism, is relevant to our purpose and will be addressed later.

The thyroid gland is a butterfly-shaped structure, with two pear-shaped lobes molded to the trachea (windpipe of the neck). Thyroid hormones, thyroxine (T_4) in particular, stimulate metabolism. Metabolism is the rate at which food is converted into heat and energy. The correct functioning of the thyroid gland requires iodine in the diet. Thus, people who do not have enough iodine develop iodine deficiency goiter, a swelling of the thyroid (visible on the neck), which results in underactivity of the thyroid. Underactivity of the thyroid is called hypothyroidism. This disorder has a number of psychiatric symptoms to be addressed in detail here. At the moment, it is important to highlight the fact that the thyroid regulates metabolism. Thus, hypothyroidism entails a lowered metabolic rate—lowered body temperature, lowered heart rate, psychomotor (psychological and motoric) retardation, fatigue and lethargy, and decreased appetite, hearing, taste, and smell. Alternatively, hyperthyroidism is overactivity of the thyroid and results in a raised metabolic rate. Thus, some symptoms of hyperthyroidism are increased body temperature, faster heartbeat, difficultly sleeping and staying asleep, hyperarousal, distractibility, and overactivity. Hyperthyroidism includes a variety of psychiatric symptoms that we will describe later.

The parathyroids are four tiny glands, each about the size of a Spanish peanut or a pearl, embedded in the four corners (tips of the wings) of the butterfly-shaped thyroid gland. The parathyroids produce parathyroid hormone (or parahormone), which helps maintain plasma (blood) calcium level by working with Vitamin D and calcitonin (a hormone produced by the thyroid). Reduction or increase in parathyroid hormone changes the level of plasma calcium and results in excitability of the nerves and neuromuscular functions, convulsions, kidney stones, problems of bone development, and a wide range of psychiatric symptoms.

The pancreas is a long thin gland that lies crosswise (horizontal) just behind the stomach. Insulin (from the Latin *insula* meaning island) is produced by the pancreas, in an area called the islets or islands of Langerhans (hence the name insulin). Insulin helps the body use sugar and other carbohydrates correctly. The term *carbohydrate* refers to substances made of carbon *(carbo,)* hydrogen, and oxygen *(hydrate)* and includes sugars and starches. Insulin regulates carbohydrate metabolism and facilitates the entry of glucose (a sugar) into cells, lowering blood sugar. In a complex feedback system, our current blood sugar level itself stimulates the secretion of insulin to lower that blood sugar level to normal; when we eat several candy bars, insulin is secreted in response. However, if there is damage to the beta cells of the islands of Langerhans, inadequate amounts of insulin are secreted. This allows glucose (glycemia) to accumulate in the blood, such that one has high blood sugar (hyperglycemia) and carbohydrate metabolism is abnormal. This condition is called diabetes mellitus; thus, diabetics must restrict their intake of sugar and must inject themselves with insulin to maintain normal carbohydrate metabolism. There are many neuropsychological and psychiatric symptoms and correlates of diabetes. We will not cover diabetes here, however, because it is rarely misdiagnosed as a psychiatric disorder.

The "sort-of-opposite" of diabetes is hyperinsulinism, a condition in which the pancreas produces and secretes too much insulin. This lowers the blood sugar level considerably, resulting in a condition called hypoglycemia. Thus, hypoglycemics are often told to drink fruit juice or eat a candy bar to reestablish physiological homeostasis—balance. There is considerable debate regarding the psychiatric symptoms associated with hypoglycemia; many consider these symptoms to be a direct manifestation of the physical disorder (low blood sugar), whereas others construe this disorder to be a hoax. We will address these issues.

The adrenal glands are perched on top of each kidney, each about the size of a ripe, red grape. Each adrenal gland has two parts, (a) the medulla or core and (b) the adrenal cortex or covering. The adrenal medulla produces epinephrine (often called adrenalin from "adrenal") and norepinephrine (often called noradrenalin). Epinephrine and norepinephrine are not only hormones but also belong to a class of chemicals called *neurotransmitters.* These are the chemicals that transmit or carry messages from the body to the brain and back, as well as around the brain. Many theories suggest that changes in the levels of these two neurotransmitters in particular are related to depressive and manic symptoms. These two neurotransmitters have several other functions (e.g., they are mobilized for emergencies and other responses to stress) that are not relevant to our focus.

The adrenal cortex produces a variety of hormones, the most relevant of which are the steroids (because they are produced in the adrenal cortex, steroids are also called corticosteroids). These hormones are often called "the stress hormones" because they play complex roles in bodily reactions to physical and psychological stress. An excess or overproduction of steroids causes an endocrinological disorder called Cushing's syndrome; this disorder has a host of psychiatric, neurological, and physical symptoms. A deficit or underproduction of steroids causes an endocrinological disorder called Addison's disease, which also has several psychiatric symptoms.

Endocrinological Disorders

Most of the syndromes associated with endocrine dysfunction manifest themselves in psychological symptoms. These syndromes are easily diagnosed through blood tests, analyses of urine, or both, and most are easily treated. These endocrinological disorders tend to appear in clusters, such that, if a patient has one of these disorders, she (these disorders occur most often in women) is highly likely to develop another, related disorder; if she does not, one or several of her women family members will. Endocrinological disorders characterized by hyperactivity and hyperproduction of a hormone (hyperdisorders) typically cluster together. These clustered, related disorders are known as *multiple endocrine neoplasia syndromes,* or (ironically) MEN syndromes. Similarly, the disorders characterized by hypoactivity and hypoproduction of a hormone (hypodisorders) cluster together and are known as *polyglandular insufficiency* syndromes. The exception to this clustering rule is that hyperthyroidism clusters with the hypodisorders because after a number of years (5-20 years), hyperthyroidism typically changes into hypothyroidism (Greenspan & Forsham, 1983; Nemeroff & Loosen, 1987).

The discussions of these disorders that follow are descriptions of pure (prototypical) presentations of a single disorder. Many patients will have a cluster of these disorders and so exhibit symptoms of several disorders simultaneously.

References

Greenspan, F. S., & Forsham, P. H. (1983). *Basic and clinical endocrinology.* Los Altos, CA: Lange Medical.
Nemeroff, C. B., & Loosen, P. T. (1987). *Handbook of clinical psychoneuroendocrinology.* New York: Guilford.
Williams, R. H. (1981). *Textbook of endocrinology* (6th ed.). Philadelphia: W. B. Saunders.

Thyroid Disorders

Hyperthyroidism and Hypothyroidism

In this chapter, we focus on disorders due to overactivity or underactivity of the thyroid gland.

Thyrotoxicosis or Hyperthyroidism

This disorder results from an excess of the thyroid hormone thyroxine (T_4). If the cause is endogenous (e.g., hyperactivity of the thyroid gland), it is called *Graves' disease*. If the cause is exogenous (e.g., previous thyroid treatments), it is called *hyperthyroidism*. The cause of this disorder is unknown. In endogenous hyperthyroidism, the thyroid is hyperactive for unknown reasons. In exogenous hyperthyroidism, the cause often is previous thyroid treatments.

The major psychiatric symptoms of hyperthyroidism are shown in Table 2.1. Several other symptoms are associated and may or may not appear:

- Associated psychotic symptoms of the manic, hypomanic, or bipolar type in some cases
- Distractibility with short attention span present in most cases
- Impaired recent memory in most cases
- Attacks of diarrhea, sweating, and generalized weakness in all cases
- Increased appetite but with a loss of weight or stable weight in all cases
- Red, puffy eyelids in many cases

Obviously, the symptoms of hyperthyroidism can be difficult to distinguish from bipolar and anxiety disorders and symptoms. Hyperthyroidism

Table 2.1   Major Psychiatric Symptoms of Hyperthyroidism

Incessant tension, restlessness, and agitation
Inability to relax (the need "to do" something)
Flight of ideas
Psychomotor acceleration in the presence of chronic fatigue, tiredness, and weakness
Insomnia (typically initial insomnia, difficulty falling asleep)
Pressure of speech
Excitability and irritability
Emotional lability (with inappropriate outbursts of euphoria, anger, crying)
Tangential and circumstantial speech
Chronic, diffuse, severe anxiety (sometimes due to mitral valve prolapse, which often
  accompanies this disorder)

may be present in patients who appear to have any of the following psychiatric disorders: (a) agitated (atypical) depression, (b) bipolar disorder (depressed or manic at the time), (c) cyclothymia, or (d) generalized anxiety disorder with or without an associated dysthymic or major depressive disorder. In our experience and according to the literature (see references), hyperthyroidism is most likely to present as an atypical depression with or without an associated generalized anxiety disorder. The bipolar and manic presentations are also common, however.

To complicate the matter of this physical disorder that typically presents as depression, anxiety, or both, hyperthyroidism is also 7 times more frequent in women than in men and, indeed, typically runs in families among the women (mother, her sisters, and her daughters). Depressive and anxiety disorders also typically occur in women. Thus, an unknown but probably large percentage of depressed or anxious women may suffer from hyperthyroidism but may be misdiagnosed and mistaken as suffering from depressive or anxiety disorder—with an ostensible genetic component as a result of its familial pattern. Although far more common in women of all ethnic groups than in men, hyperthyroidism is also somewhat more frequent among African American women than among White women.

Treatment

The psychiatric symptoms seen in hyperthyroid patients *should not be treated with tricyclic antidepressants or lithium* because both of these exacerbate rather than decrease the symptoms. The patient gets worse because of the "increased toxicity . . . probably due to the increased sensitivity to catecholamines that exists in these patients" (Morley & Krahn, 1987, p. 18), and therefore appears to be deteriorating and incurable. Likewise, these psychiatric symptoms *should not be treated with antipsychotics* (e.g., Haldol, Mellaril) because these drugs also exacerbate the symptoms and the increased toxicity they create in hyperthyroid patients can lead to fatal dystonic reactions. Unfortunately, once misdiagnosed as having bipolar, generalized anxiety or depressive disorder, hyperthyroid patients are often prescribed these drugs because they are the acceptable pharmacological treatment (under ordinary circumstances) for these psychiatric symptoms. The hyperthyroid patient, however, is not a psychiatric patient despite her symptoms. Rather, the hyperthyroid patient has a physical disorder known to cause these symptoms. The therapy of choice is to treat that physical disorder with medication for thyroid dysfunction; treating the symptoms as if they are psychiatric in origin (with therapy, psychotropic medications, or both) is misguided and dangerous.

Differential Diagnosis

The last few symptoms of hyperthyroidism (diarrhea; increased appetite with weight loss; red, puffy eyelids) are fairly reliable physical symptoms typically not associated with bipolar disorder, anxiety, or depression. Alertness to these may assist in differentiating hyperthyroidism from a psychiatric disorder. Women (particularly African American women) who present any of the psychiatric symptoms here to a therapist should routinely be questioned about these physical, differential diagnostic signs of hyperthyroidism. In addition, *all* women presenting such psychiatric symptoms should be questioned about the recency of their last physical exam and whether it included a "thyroid panel." This is a simple blood test for thyroid dysfunction that can easily be run on the blood drawn in the course of a routine physical. Unfortunately, however, the patient often must ask for it to be run. If a woman seeking therapy and displaying these symptoms has not had a physical recently (within the past 6 months and including a thyroid panel) or has not had a recent thyroid panel, the prudent course of action would be to request that the patient have this done immediately. A routine thyroid panel can be run on a small sample of blood drawn from the patient for this purpose at any hospital, including emergency rooms. Patients needn't have excellent or even adequate medical insurance to have this quick, inexpensive test.

Subclinical Hyperthyroidism

In addition, a subacute or subclinical (milder) form of hyperthyroidism is suspected to be rampant in the general population of women and is known to be caused by *repeated, ordinary viral infections.* This form of the disorder often (but not always) involves pain in the thyroid gland (reported as a lump in the throat or the sensation of being strangled—this dismissed as hysteria or histrionics) and is associated with mild symptoms of either or both hyperthyroidism and hypothyroidism.

Aging and Hyperthyroidism

Finally, a subset of aged, hyperthyroid patients will exhibit severe depression, with extreme apathy and withdrawal, in a manner indistinguishable from a major depressive episode; anxiety, agitation, and bipolar symptoms are absent. This form of hyperthyroidism is called *apathetic thyrotoxicosis* and is a disorder of concern in geriatric women who exhibit symptoms of extreme depression.

Hypothyroidism

This disorder results from underactivity of the thyroid gland (less output than normal) due to hypothalamic, pituitary, or thyroid disease. Hypothyroidism develops very slowly over time, with mild symptoms present and increasing in number and severity for many years. Thus, the disorder typically is not recognized by patient, family, or physician until it is well advanced. It is far more common among women than among men. The major symptoms of hypothyroidism are as follows:

- *Generalized psychomotor retardation,* in which all cognitive and behavioral activities are slowed down: There is decreased initiative, slow speech, impaired short- and long-term memory, impaired concentration, and marked slowness in comprehension.
- *Fatigue and weakness* that are generalized and severe and associated with a host of minor aches and pains (mild, multiple somatic complaints): Patients are so chronically tired, slowed down, and "worn out" that they cannot complete the simplest tasks. This fatigue is often associated with complaints of drowsiness.
- *Depression* that is insidious in its onset, has been present for several years (perhaps as long as the patient can remember) but has been slowly increasing in severity: The severely depressed mood is accompanied by feelings of hopeless-

ness, suicidal ideation, frequent crying spells, anhedonia, and hypersomnia. Typically, poverty of speech is present. In a few patients, episodic irritability, insomnia, and depersonalization also may appear.

- *Associated symptoms,* including complaints of always feeling cold and of tingling and numbness in the fingers (called peripheral neuropathy): Patients may also complain of headaches, weakness, not hearing well, fatigue, loss of appetite (*with weight gain*), constipation, stiff and aching muscles, and excessive and irregular menstrual bleeding. In time, their eyes are puffy and their hair becomes dry and brittle and may fall out.

Clearly, the hypothyroid patient appears to suffer from a major depressive episode. The patient is disheveled, cries a lot, is suicidal, and complains of depression. She exhibits psychomotor retardation, appetite loss, anhedonia, hypersomnia, and multiple, vague somatic complaints and preoccupations. Because the patient appears to be suffering from a prototypical major depressive episode, it is extremely difficult to differentiate this physical disorder from a psychiatric disorder.

Test Scores

On psychological and neuropsychological tests, the hypothyroid patient exhibits signs of impaired abstraction, memory, and concentration. Low scores on the Wechsler Adult Intelligence Scale (WAIS) Digit Span, Vocabulary, and Block Design typically are found, along with impaired scores on the Halstead-Reitan Trailmaking Test. On the Minnesota Multiphasic Personality Inventory (MMPI), a pattern of clinically significant elevations on Scales 2, 6, 7, and 8 are seen, these again suggesting a psychotic depression; however, her scores on all of the other subscales of the MMPI will also be elevated and typically in the $T = 60$ to 65 range. We use *she* again because this disorder is far more common among women than among men and is typically seen in women between the ages of 40 and 60—the ages when the symptoms are most severe.

Treatment and Differential Diagnosis

Like the hyperthyroid patient, the hypothyroid patient *cannot be treated with antidepressants, lithium, or antipsychotics.* These drugs, often used to treat such symptoms, exacerbate them. Patients who take them show a rapid deterioration in response to such psychotropic agents and therefore appear to be deteriorating and incurable. Hypothyroid patients are cured only by thyroid hormone replacement therapy. For such therapy to be initiated, however, the disorder must be accurately diagnosed. Alertness to the physical symptoms of hypothyroidism can assist in differentiating it from a major depressive episode. These symptoms typically do not appear in major depressive episodes and are (a) dry skin; (b) dry, brittle hair that falls out; (c) constipation; (d) weight gain despite appetite loss; (e) cold intolerance; (f) hoarseness; and (g) hearing loss. Like hyperthyroidism, this disorder is readily diagnosed by a simple blood test.

A Case Example: Anna

Anna is a 49-year-old, White sociologist who has been a professor in the sociology department of a major university for the past 20 years. She is well-known for her research on women and is considered a valued, but "eccentric," faculty member. For the past 10 years, her colleagues and students (her research assistants in particular) have become increasingly concerned about her mental health. Students report that Anna either appears in her classes on time, well prepared and delivering a brilliant lecture, or simply fails to appear at all. In her classes and in faculty meetings, she is either brilliant and perceptive or disorganized, tangential, confused, disheveled, exhausted, and bizarre. The chair of her department often says of her, "When Anna steps to the podium in her classroom and opens her bag, you never know if she's gonna pull out a book or a chicken." On the many occasions that Anna fails to appear for her scheduled lecture or a departmental meeting, she is often discovered sitting in her office, staring out the window, complaining of fatigue and apparently unaware of her scheduled class, or she's found wandering the halls of the department, with her dry, brittle gray hair sticking up (earning her the nickname, "the witch"), her slip down to her knees, and mayonnaise on her nose, apparently unaware of where she's supposed to be and of what she looks like. Her research assistants complain that she doesn't seem to remember things she's said or done or recall meetings she's scheduled with them and that they have been carrying the load for her research for months.

This odd behavior was tolerated by many of her colleagues and labeled eccentric rather than disturbed, in part because of the excellence of her work and her reputation, in part because labeling her as disturbed meant that they would have to do something about her, and sadly, in part because her oddities provided a source of amusement for everyone. Anna's colleagues ceased regarding her as "eccentric and charming" and became concerned about her when her fatigue seemed to increase and disrupted her ability to teach and when she began to exhibit symptoms of severe depression in addition to the afore-mentioned episodic confused state. More and more frequently, Anna would appear in the department late, tired, tearful, and confused, only to discover that she had left vital materials (e.g., her lecture, an exam) at home—a place that her colleagues all too often found with the doors left open and unlocked. Finally, Anna seemed to be losing her hearing; she either did not respond to questions or requested that people speak louder and had herself begun to shout in a hoarse voice. Feeling uncomfortable about questioning Anna regarding what appeared to be dementia but nonetheless concerned for her, Anna's colleagues confronted her about the least disturbing of her symptoms—namely, her inability to hear and her shouting. Her colleagues suggested only that she have her hearing checked. This was the least serious of her symptoms but was the only one that her colleagues felt comfortable mentioning.

Within a week of this suggestion, Anna had her hearing checked and was found to have no primary hearing disorder. She then had a complete physical, and severe hypothyroidism was discovered. After several months of thyroid replacement therapy, Anna's behavior improved considerably. Although still eccentric and prone to memory lapses, Anna no longer displays symptoms of severe depression, lethargy, or generalized mental confusion. Her hair remains dry and brittle and falls out.

Unlike many women, Anna never sought therapy for her symptoms, including her symptoms of depression. Had she done so, however, it is likely that she would have been misperceived as a woman suffering from a depression caused by her divorce and conflicts with her adult children; her hearing loss, confusion, and dry, brittle hair no doubt would have been dismissed as irrelevant symptoms. Once misperceived as a woman suffering from depression, Anna may have been prescribed tricyclic antidepressants whose effects would have been lethal. Ironically, then, Anna's colleagues' inordinate discomfort with confronting her about anything save her apparent hearing loss led her to focus on a physical symptom and seek the medical tests that inevitably resulted in the accurate diagnosis of hypothyroidism. Had her colleagues been less timid and confronted her instead about her depression, memory lapses, and periods of confusion, she would have sought psychiatric help that could have resulted in a psychiatric misdiagnosis and subsequent dangerous or lethal treatment; as discussed later, treating the symptoms of hypothyroidism with antidepressant drugs can result in a woman's death.

Even when the physical diagnosis has been correctly made, the ostensible psychiatric nature of some of the symptoms of hypothyroidism can remain problematic, as indicated in the next case.

A Case Example: Thelma

Thelma is a 37-year-old African American woman who presented herself to a therapist because of long-standing feelings of depression. During the routine physically oriented questions the therapist asked as part of the intake interview, Thelma revealed that she had been diagnosed as having hypothyroidism many years ago. Her physician merely informed her that she had a thyroid disorder and initiated treatment of it without informing her of the psychiatric symptoms involved in the disorder and without asking her any specific questions about these. Thelma, having no idea that her psychiatric symptoms were related to her thyroid dysfunction and not wishing to "bother" her doctor with a psychiatric complaint, did not reveal these symptoms to her physician; her physician, consequently, did not know that some of the symptoms (the psychiatric ones) of her thyroid disorder were not yet under complete control and so could not titrate her treatment to control these symptoms. Instead of talking to her physician, Thelma spent several years seeking psychotherapy from a number of different practitioners, none of whom had been able to alleviate her depression through psychotherapy.

Thus, Thelma had been depressed for many years without knowing that these feelings were the result of hypothyroidism that was not fully controlled by her current medical treatments for that disorder. The therapist explained to Thelma the relationship between her physical disorder and depression and suggested that Thelma return to her physician and reveal these symptoms to acquire additional treatment for the thyroid disorder, their most likely cause. The therapist also suggested that, if after receiving additional treatment for thyroid dysfunction, Thelma remained depressed nonetheless, she should return for treatment for that depression. Thelma's physician was then called and the depression discussed with him. Her physician was not aware of her depression and made an appointment with Thelma to reevaluate her thyroid dysfunction.

Thus, as discussed in the Introduction, many women (and many therapists) immediately categorize symptoms as physical or as psychiatric, and that categorization can be an error. Thelma categorized her symptoms of tiredness, lethargy, coldness, appetite loss, weight gain, and hearing loss as "physical"; she sought treatment from her physician for these symptoms alone and was diagnosed as having hypothyroidism. She did not at any time, however, reveal her depression to her physician because she believed this symptom to be "psychiatric"—unrelated to her physical symptoms and physical disorder and appropriate to discuss only with a therapist. Consequently, in repeated visits with her physician, when asked if she was having any problems or symptoms, Thelma had answered that she had none, so her physician had not altered her medical treatment. Thelma's case reveals that the accurate diagnosis and treatment of women require not only that psychotherapists ask women questions about their physical symptoms and consider physical disorders a possibility but also that they *encourage women to discuss psychiatric symptoms with physicians.* Only both steps obstruct the problems that can ensue from the tendency to assume that certain types of symptoms are physical and others are psychiatric in origin; all symptoms can probably be classified into either of these categories.

Myxedema Madness

If hypothyroidism is misdiagnosed and therefore not treated with hormone replacement therapy, a severe psychosis with symptoms of dementia is likely to result. That is, if the patient's true condition is untreated as a result of psychiatric misdiagnosis, additional and more severe psychiatric symptoms appear. This psychosis is called *myxedema* (sometimes called myxedema madness). This syndrome is characterized by a general deterioration of all cognitive functions, extreme paranoid ideation, and auditory hallucinations; it is indistinguishable from paranoid schizophrenia, with the exception that it suddenly appears in a patient who had appeared to be depressed. If the hypothyroid patient is elderly, myxedema madness is likely to be misdiagnosed as senile dementia.

(Ostensible) Rapid-Cycling Bipolar Disorder

In addition to presenting as a major depression, schizophrenia, or dementia, hypothyroidism has other faces as well. Several clinicians and researchers have found that clinical and subclinical hypothyroidism can present in symptoms indistinguishable from a rapid-cycling, bipolar disorder, in which patients have at least four episodes of mania and of depression per year. This cycling can be from normal mood to depression and back or from depression to mania and back. This rapid-cycling (ostensible) bipolar disorder is often iatrogenic—caused by being treated with lithium or antidepressants for what was mistaken to be cyclothymia or dysthymia. That is, because the onset of hypothyroidism is insidious, patients often seek treatment from therapists early in the disorder when their symptoms are mild. The standard pharmacological treatment for a mild depression or for cyclothymia (antidepressants or lithium) then precipitates a rapid-cycling, bizarre, apparently bipolar disorder (see Cowdry et al., 1983, for an explanation of the physiology of why). Subclinical hypothyroid patients are those who test normally on one but not on the other blood tests for the disorder. These patients also fail to exhibit the differential diagnostic physical symptoms (dry skin, weight gain, constipation, cold intolerance, fatigue, hoarseness). Thus, the subclinical form of the disorder is particularly likely to be misdiagnosed as an affective disorder, to be treated with antidepressants, and to therefore result in an iatrogenic, rapid-cycling bipolar-like disorder.

As a result of being untreated for several years, hypothyroidism can result in a delirium with or without psychotic symptoms, which can and often does lead to coma and death. *Women can and do die* prematurely and unnecessarily, during years of useless psychotherapy, from the misdiagnosis of physical disorders as psychiatric. The importance of these misdiagnoses cannot possibly be overemphasized.

Irrespective of whether the hypothyroid patient's symptoms are depressive, schizophrenic, demented, delirious, or bipolar, these symptoms are cured

Table 2.2 Comparing Hyperthyroidism and Hypothyroidism

Hyperthyroidism	*Hypothyroidism*
Increased appetite	Decreased appetite
Weight loss or stable	Weight gain
Heat intolerance	Cold intolerance
Tachycardia (rapid heartbeat)	Bradycardia (slowed heartbeat)
Diarrhea	Constipation
Mania, anxiety, psychomotor acceleration	Depression, anhedonia, psychomotor retardation
Insomnia	Hypersomnia

by thyroid hormone replacement therapy; 3 months of this treatment may be necessary before improvement is shown and symptoms begin to subside. Lithium, antipsychotics, benzodiazepines, antidepressants, and sedative hypnotics can cause hypothyroidism and exacerbate preexisting clinical or subclinical hypothyroidism. Lithium, in particular, is notorious for precipitating hypothyroidism. Dilantin and barbiturates have also been reported to cause hypothyroidism.

Aging and Hypothyroidism

Many of the endocrinological changes associated with aging involve a decrease in certain hormones, and therefore, deficiency or hypodisorders such as hypothyroidism and diabetes (deficient insulin), may be seen. Awareness of these endocrinological changes can assist in differentiating hypothyroidism in elderly women from dementia, depression, and schizophrenia.

Summary

Hyperthyroidism and hypothyroidism present in nearly opposite constellations of symptoms, with the exception that both can present depressive symptoms. The symptoms of these two disorders are compared in Table 2.2.

These two disorders are common, common in women (and in African Americans), and easily misdiagnosed as psychiatric. Once misdiagnosed, these patients are then often treated with all "the right" pharmacological and psychotherapeutic interventions for a psychiatric disorder that the patients do not have. The patients therefore show no improvement in treatment, and that often leads to increasing the treatment (e.g., the dosage of lithium or antidepressants). This aggressive treatment, as well as the failure to treat the disorder the patient actually has, then elicits additional symptoms and leads to patient deterioration or death. This unfortunate sequence of events is the logical and frequent outcome of assuming that depressed and anxious women necessarily have psychiatric disorders. As we shall see, this sequence is prototypical of responses to a diversity of other physical disorders.

References

Cowdry, R., Wehr, T., et al. (1983). Thyroid abnormalities associated with rapid-cycling bipolar illness. *Archives of General Psychiatry, 46,* 414-420.

Morley, J. E., & Krahn, D. D. (1987). Endocrinology for the psychiatrist. In C. B. Nemeroff & Loosen (Eds.), *Handbook of clinical psychoneuroendocrinology* (pp. 3-37). New York: Guilford.

Adrenal, Pituitary, and Parathyroid Disorders

In this chapter, we discuss disorders resulting from abnormal activity of the adrenal, pituitary, and parathyroid glands.

Adrenal Disorders

Addison's disease occurs when the production of steroid hormones by the adrenal cortex gradually decreases over the years. The most common cause is that the body (the immunological system that fights viruses and bacteria) attacks the adrenal cortex because it mistook it for an invading virus, bacterium, or foreign agent; the reasons that the body does this are unknown. When the body attacks itself in this manner, the disorder is called *an autoimmune disorder;* Addison's disease is an autoimmune disorder.

The steady decrease in all circulating corticosteroids over a period of many years is so slow that Addison's disease is neither recognized nor diagnosed as such until late in the disease. The psychiatric symptoms of the disease are present from the beginning, however, and are typically misdiagnosed as psychogenic in origin. They include

- apathy,
- fatigue,
- lack of initiative,
- depression (chronic depressive mood),
- poverty of thought,

- social withdrawal,
- psychomotor retardation, and
- recent memory impairment.

In addition, patients also present chronic tiredness and weakness and loss of appetite with weight loss. There may also be nausea, vomiting, and weakness in its early stages, along with a craving for salt. In later stages, there is a frank psychosis with hallucinations, delusions, and thought disorder.

Given its insidious, slow onset, Addison's disease is usually misdiagnosed as depression until very late in the disease when there is a darkening of pigmentation that acts as a differential diagnostic sign (and remains after treatment). During the earlier stages of the disease, there are no major differential diagnostic signs except the craving for salt and nausea and vomiting, which are not present in all cases. Thus, depressed women should be questioned about their salt intake and about nausea and vomiting, and Addison's disease should be considered a possibility in all cases of depression. It can be diagnosed through a routine urine test, something that should be conducted to rule out physical disorders in all patients.

Cushing's syndrome results from a chronic excess of circulating cortisol (one of the steroids). The most common causes are hypothalamic dysfunction or adrenal disease. The psychological symptoms of Cushing's syndrome generally precede the physical symptoms; serious psychiatric problems appear in 50% of Cushing patients.

The primary psychological symptoms of this disease are severe depression with intense suicidal ideation and high risk of suicide. The associated symptoms are

- insomnia,
- loss of libido,
- irritability,
- loss of recent memory, and
- difficulty concentrating.

Manic excitement and euphoria do not occur. However, there are periods of acute anxiety, agitation, and emotional lability.

Once again, the major symptoms of an endocrinological disorder are prototypically depressive ones; this disease, like the many others discussed thus far, must be considered a possible cause of depressive symptoms in women.

Cushing's syndrome has a few other faces as well. Although the majority of people with the disease exhibit depressive symptoms, approximately 15%

of cases will present in a prototypical paranoid or depressive psychosis that includes paranoid or depressive delusions and associated hallucinations. In addition, when the cause of Cushing's syndrome is exogenous corticosteroids (e.g., voluntary abuse of steroids or use of steroids to fight a severe illness), the symptoms are different. In these cases, 75% of patients show euphoria, increased activity level, decreased need for sleep, increased appetite, and increased libido. Although the symptoms in these patients are on the "high" side of normal, the majority do not meet the criteria for mania (e.g., they do not exhibit pressure of speech, flight of ideas, expansiveness, or psychotic symptoms). A small percentage, however, do exhibit symptoms of a manic psychosis.

The physical symptoms of Cushing's syndrome can aid in differential diagnosis but, unfortunately, do not appear until late in the disease. These include weight gain, facial obesity, hypertension, muscle wasting, and amenorrhea. Cushing's syndrome tends to occur in women (and sometimes men) ages 20 to 60 and has no preference for a specific ethnic group.

Pituitary Disorders

Hypopituitarism results when a tumor, lesion, infection, or severe head injury destroys a portion of the pituitary gland. Because this gland sends chemical messages to the adrenals, thyroid, and other target glands, pituitary disorders entail the symptoms of both thyroid and adrenal dysfunctions. Psychological symptoms are always present in hypopituitarism. The most common symptoms are

- profound apathy and indifference,
- inactivity,
- fatigue,
- depression,
- loss of libido,
- drowsiness,
- dependent behavior, and
- severe, *extreme* loss of appetite and weight.

Hypopituitarism is readily misdiagnosed as a prototypical severe or psychotic depression, with dependent personality disorder and anorexia nervosa (the weight loss is so extreme that it meets the criteria for anorexia).

As with other endocrinological disorders, late in this disorder, specific physical symptoms appear that assist in differentiating it from psychopathology:

- waxy skin,
- fine wrinkles around the mouth and eyes that give the patient the appearance of premature aging,
- loss of body hair,
- loss of pigmentation of the nipples, and
- inability to tan.

Parathyroid Disorders

Hypoparathyroidism—Hypocalcemia

In this syndrome, the parathyroid glands fail to produce enough of their hormones, which leads to a decrease in serum calcium. Its two common causes are (a) thyroid operations that disrupt parathyroid functions and (b) vitamin D deficiency that is secondary to nutritional deficiency or kidney disorders. This disorder rarely occurs in adults. It is found instead in children, and in girls far more often than in boys. It includes the following psychiatric symptoms:

- depression,
- emotional lability,
- anxiety, and
- irritability and fatigue.

Thus, this disorder is readily misdiagnosed as a depressive or anxiety disorder in female children and teenagers. If left untreated, it progresses, and several physical symptoms appear that assist in differentiating it from childhood psychopathology. These symptoms are tingling and numbness in the face and hands; frequent headaches; seizures with convulsions; poor tooth development; childhood mental retardation; thin, patchy hair; muscular weakness; and painful cramplike spasms in the hands, feet, and throat (this last symptom is called *tetany*).

This disorder is readily treated with calcium and Vitamin D supplements and is easily diagnosed through blood tests. In the absence of those tests, however, hypoparathyroidism can be misdiagnosed as any number of disorders, ranging from epilepsy and brain tumors to mental retardation and anxiety and depressive disorders. Thin, patchy hair and tetany are differential diagnostic features but, unfortunately, do not appear until very late in the disease, often after the girl has been misdiagnosed as having a psychiatric disorder.

Hyperparathyroidism—Hypercalcemia

This syndrome is the result of excessive amounts of parathyroid hormones that lead to increased serum levels of calcium. The most common causes of this syndrome are (a) a benign tumor on one of the four parathyroid glands and (b) hypervitaminosis D (excessive intake of Vitamin D). It is rare before puberty and instead tends to appear in adults, where it is 2 to 3 times more common among women than among men. In the early stages of hypercalcemia, the presenting symptoms are purely psychological and behavioral and consist of a constellation of vague, "neurotic" symptoms that do not clearly fit any well-defined category in the *Diagnostic and Statistical Manual of Mental Disorders (DSM)*. These include

- depression with suicidal tendencies,
- chronic and severe anxiety,
- lack of initiative and spontaneity, and
- symptoms of any of the personality disorders (depending on the patient).

In later stages, symptoms include confusion, loss of concentration, and marked short-term memory defects, all of which increase the chances of the disorder's being misdiagnosed as a depressive disorder, anxiety disorder, or both.

The physical symptoms of hypercalcemia *do not assist* in differentiating it from psychological disorders but, rather, increase the number of psychiatric disorders for which it can be mistaken. These physical symptoms include

- dull back pain,
- frequent urinary tract infections,
- gastrointestinal dysfunctions, including nausea, vomiting, and constipation, and
- abdominal pain.

These physical symptoms are readily misdiagnosed as the typical somatic complaints seen in a depressive or anxiety disorder, or they can be misunderstood and misdiagnosed as hypochondriasis, somatization disorder, affective disorder, personality disorder, or anxiety disorder. Like the other disorders we've discussed, it is readily diagnosed correctly through simple, inexpensive blood tests.

Summary

Endocrinological disorders can be misdiagnosed as psychiatric disorders because their major symptoms are depressive, anxiety, or bipolar symptoms. Treating these disorders as if they are functional (psychiatric, social) in origin by prescribing lithium, antidepressants, or antianxiety agents can exacerbate the symptoms. Furthermore, the use of these and other psychotropic medications in some cases causes endocrinological disorders. Thus, countless cases of ostensible depression, anxiety disorder, anorexia nervosa, personality disorder, and bipolar disorder among women and girls may actually be misdiagnosed endocrine dysfunction because (a) endocrinological disorders occur far more often in women than in men and (b) therapists rarely rule out these disorders before rendering psychiatric verdicts. The need to assess for these disorders as a routine aspect of clinical practice is clear and is essential to the health and welfare of women. Research is also needed on the extent to which misdiagnosed endocrinological disorders account for women's high rate of (ostensible) anxiety and depressive disorders as well as for gender differences in the prevalence of those.

We turn now to seizure disorders and their many psychiatric presentations.

PART II

Seizure Disorders

Introduction to Seizure Disorders

The cells of the brain communicate with each other by sending tiny electrical signals back and forth. Epilepsy exists whenever a group of cells sends signals that are too strong, are too weak, or deviate from the normal shape and speed. These sudden, abnormal electrical discharges in the brain are called seizures. *Seizures refer to events in the brain* and not to behaviors or convulsions. The behavioral signs and manifestations of a seizure vary with the precise brain area in which the abnormal discharge occurs.

For example, if the seizure occurs in the portions of the brain that control movement (or across the entire brain so that the areas that control movement are affected), then convulsions (bodily jerking) are often the behavioral manifestation of the seizure. As we will see, however, the most common types of seizures are localized to portions of the brain that control language, emotion, and memory; these seizures manifest themselves, not in convulsions, but in depression, anxiety, hallucinations, lost time, and other apparently psychiatric symptoms and disorders.

Technically, a seizure is defined as *a transient, paroxysmal, pathophysiological disturbance of brain function caused by a spontaneous, excessive discharge of cortical neurons,* whose symptoms are contingent on the nature and location of the discharge. In the normal adult, the electrical signals used by the cells of the brain to communicate are 8 to 13 cycles per second (cps); these are called alpha waves. Abnormal electrical discharges may be too fast (more than 13 cps, called beta waves) or too slow (4-7 cps, called theta waves), or extremely slow (0.5-3.5 cps, called delta waves). The precise symptoms shown by any individual vary by type of seizure pattern (there are many others) and the location in the brain of the abnormal discharge.

Epilepsy is a chronic condition characterized by recurrent seizures. Epilepsy is not itself a disease but is instead a symptom of some other brain or physiological disturbance. Seizures are measured and diagnosed through an electroencephalogram (EEG) test, in which electrodes are placed in various spots on the surface of the head to measure the electrical activity of the brain.[1]

Stages of a Seizure

For many kinds of seizures, different symptoms are shown during the various phases or stages of the seizure. A seizure can be conceptualized as having five distinct stages:

1. *A prodromal stage,* the hours or days before the seizure.
2. *A primictal stage,* the minutes just before *(prim)* the seizure *(ictal).*
3. *An ictal stage,* the period of the seizure.
4. *A postictal stage,* the minutes and hours just after *(post)* the seizure
5. *An interictal stage,* the weeks or months between seizures.

Causes of Seizures

Seizures are sometimes classified as either primary or secondary, with these terms referring to the cause rather than the type of seizure. Like the endocrinological disorders, *primary seizure disorders* refer to those that appear to be genetic or endogenous; usually, these are seizures of the generalized type. *Secondary seizure disorders* are most likely to be caused by environmental events, prenatal events, or both; tend to be congenital; and are often of the focal or partial type (although some generalized seizures are secondary seizures). Causes of these include, but are not limited to, brain tumors (35%-40% of all people with tumors have seizures); head trauma; vascular disease; infectious diseases; anoxia at birth in particular; hypoglycemia or other disorders of glucose metabolism; toxins (poisons), such as lead or arsenic; alcohol and drug use or abuse (marijuana and LSD in particular); birth injury; and prolonged high fevers in infancy. Thus, a person whose delivery was very difficult and involved anoxia, and who then was sick as an infant and experienced a fever of 102°F or higher for at least an hour, could have a seizure disorder throughout childhood and adulthood as a result. The adult may not know that he or she has a seizure disorder if the seizures are

Table 4.1a International Classification of Epileptic Seizures

Generalized seizures
Absences (petit mal)
Myoclonus
Infantile
Clonic
Tonic
Tonic-clonic (grand mal)
Atonic
Akinetic
Partial (focal) seizures
With elementary symptoms
Motor symptoms
Sensory symptoms
Autonomic symptoms
Compound forms
With complex symptoms (psychomotor/temporal lobe epilepsy)
Impairment in consciousness only
Cognitive symptoms
Affective symptoms
Psychosensory symptoms
Psychomotor symptoms
Compound forms
Unilateral seizures
Unclassified seizures

located in the portions of the brain that control emotion and if the only symptom of the seizures is chronic depression, chronic anxiety, or episodic lost time.

Classification of Seizures

Seizures are classified in terms of the *clinical features* of the seizure and the *location* of the discharge. The standard classification system is shown in Tables 4.1a and 4.1b. As shown, seizures are usually classified into two general types: (a) *generalized seizures,* which involve widespread areas of the brain, and (b) *focal or partial seizures,* which involve only part of the brain. Although many of the seizure disorders described here are unlikely to be misdiagnosed as psychopathology, some are quite likely to be, and one type, complex *partial seizure disorder* (temporal lobe epilepsy), is highly likely to be misdiagnosed as psychopathology and so is treated in detail in Chapter 6.

Table 4.1b Further Classification of Elementary Partial and Complex Partial Seizures

Elementary Focal Seizures	Brain Localization of Discharge
Seizures with motoric symptoms	
Focal	Frontal lobe
With Jacksonian march	Precentral gyrus
Adversive	Premotor area
Postural	Supplementary motor area
Seizures with sensory symptoms	
Somatosensory	Postcentral gyrus
Visual	Occipital lobe
Auditory	Superior temporal gyrus
Vertiginous	Superior temporal gyrus
Seizures with autonomic symptoms	
Autonomic	Periinsular or fronto-temporal

Complex Partial Seizures (temporal lobe seizures)	Brain Localization of Discharge
Impairment of consciousness only	
Cognitive (thought and perception)	
Affective (mood and emotion)	
Psychosensory	
With visual hallucinations	Posterior temporal
With auditory hallucinations	Superior temporal
With olfactory hallucinations	Uncus
With gustatory hallucinations	Periinsular
With visceral hallucinations	
Psychomotor	
With automatisms	
With masticatory movements	
With speech automatisms	
With dysphasia	Dominant temporal

SOURCE: Adapted from "Clinical and Electroencephalographical Classification of Epileptic Seizures," by H. Gastaut, 1970, *Epilepsia, 11*, 102. Adapted with permission.

Kate, the woman described in the Introduction, suffered from temporal lobe epilepsy.

Because different portions of the brain control different behaviors, the kinds of symptoms seen in seizure disorders depend on precisely where in the brain the abnormal discharge is located. Thus, we turn briefly to a description of the brain's areas and the behaviors controlled by those areas before continuing this discussion of seizure disorders. The study of the behaviors, emotions, and skills controlled by various parts of the brain is typically called *localization* (specific brain area) *of function* (behavior, skill, emotion controlled by that area).

Note

1. If the results of an EEG test are positive, the person has a seizure disorder. If the results of this test are negative, however, we do not know whether the person has a seizure disorder. The problem is that for the result to be positive, the person being tested must have a seizure *during the test,* and this may not occur.

Often then, the EEG involves procedures to stress the brain to force a seizure to occur during the test. These procedures include doing the test while the person is asleep (called a "sleep recording"), because some kinds of seizures tend to occur during sleep. Alternatively, the EEG can be done after forcing the person to stay awake for 24 hours (called a *sleep-deprived EEG*), because many seizures occur when the person is fatigued. Other procedures include having the person hyperventilate (because decreasing the oxygen to the brain can force the seizure to appear), flashing a strobe light in the person's eyes (called *photic driving* or *photic stimulation*), or placing the electrodes (called "leads") in the person's nose to tap seizures that are deep in the brain (in the temporal lobes) rather than near the surface. Still, however, a person may not have a seizure during the test. Thus, a positive EEG is conclusive and a negative EEG is inconclusive.

Brain Anatomy and Localization of Function

The brain is a collection of cells and fibers inside the skull. It becomes the spinal cord as it leaves the skull. The term *central nervous system* (CNS) refers to the brain and spinal cord. The CNS is bilaterally symmetrical; most structures are duplicated on both sides of the body. Most of the CNS is also crossed or *contralateral in control.* Neurological structures on one side of the brain control body functions or parts on the opposite side. Thus, for example, the right side of the brain controls the left side of the body and vice versa. Every section of the brain works together in each action or activity. However, each section is also highly specialized and plays a different role in various functions and actions.

The brain has two sides, called *hemispheres,* that differ somewhat in the functions they control. If we could look down at our brains from above, we would see that the two hemispheres are separated by the corpus callosum; this is a structure consisting of many nerve fibers that interconnect the two hemispheres. The left hemisphere specializes in language functions and sequential reasoning or analysis (i.e., things that must be done in a series of steps, such as math) and appears to specialize in linear, causal processing of information. The right side specializes primarily in visual-spatial functions, visual analysis and synthesis (ability to recognize and understand what one sees), simultaneous or nonlinear information processing (understanding pictures, sounds, tones of voice), and a variety of emotions.

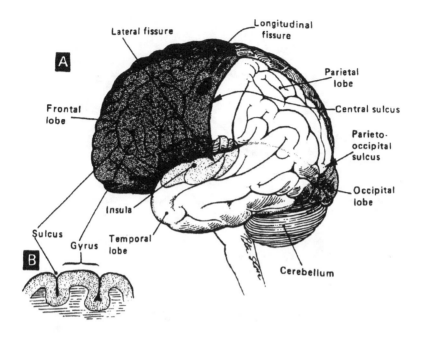

Figure 5.1. Major Fissures and Sulci

SOURCE: From *Dynamic Anatomy and Physiology* (4th ed.), by L. L. Langley, J. R. Telford, and J. B. Christensen, 1974, p. 229, St. Louis, MO: Mosby Year Book, Inc. Reprinted with permission.

Brain Structures

The term *cerebral cortex* (or *cortical)* refers to the outer covering of the brain. It is composed of neurons about 2 mm thick. Much of the cortex is contained in sulci or fissures; these are deep folds in the cortical surface. We use these fissures or sulci to divide the various areas or regions of the brain. *The central fissure* or *fissure of Rolando* divides the brain into its anterior and posterior halves. The anterior cortex lies in front of the central fissure and can be further divided into precentral and frontal areas. Pictures of the brain and its areas are shown in Figures 5.1 and 5.2.

The frontal lobe extends from the front (forehead, anterior tip) of your head to the precentral cortex. It refers to everything anterior to the Rolandic fissure. Its various areas control different functions. Area 4 is the most posterior portion of the frontal lobe. It is called the motor area because it controls volitional movement on the opposite side of the body. Disruption of

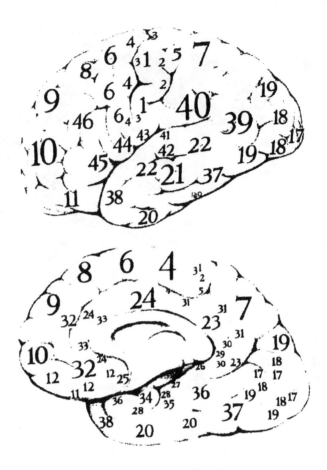

Figure 5.2. Brodman Areas

SOURCE: From *The Human Nervous System: Introduction and Review* (4th ed.), by C. R. Noback, N. L.

Area 4 causes contralateral weakness or paralysis. Area 6 is just anterior to Area 4 and is called the premotor area. It controls more complex volitional motor functions, such as taking a step up or bending a finger down on the opposite side of the body. Lesions here result in contralateral weakness or paralysis.

Area 8 is the frontal motor eye field and is anterior to the premotor area. It controls volitional eye movement. A lesion here results in ipsilateral deviation of the eyes. Area 44 is the motor-speech area and is anterior and inferior to (below) the motor and premotor area in the left hemisphere. It is called Broca's area and controls expressive speech. Areas 4, 6, 8, 9, and 10 together control contralateral smooth and skeletal muscle movement. Disturbance here results in contralateral ataxia. Areas 4, 6, 8, 9, 24, and 25 together connect to the basil ganglia (discussed later in this chapter) and play a role in complex movements of a variety of types. For example, multiple sclerosis (which occurs almost solely in White women and has many psychiatric symptoms covered later in this book) involves disruption of these areas and is characterized by ataxia.

Areas 8, 9, 10, 45, 46, and 47 are called the frontal association areas and are in the most anterior portion of the frontal lobe. This prefrontal or frontal association area appears to govern higher intellectual functions, such as the plans for all actions. For example, deciding to place a cup on the counter, pick up the coffee pot, pour coffee into the cup, and replace the pot on its burner is a highly complex plan and is under the control of the prefrontal-frontal association area. A lesion in this area (due to a car accident or Alzheimer's disease, for example) disrupts such plans; consequently, the patient might pour the coffee on the counter and then put the cup down. In addition, this prefrontal-frontal association area appears to inhibit emotional responses and to *initiate and inhibit psychomotor activity*. Thus, lesions here result not only in a disruption of the plans for behavior but also in the inability to initiate or stop an action, psychomotor retardation or hyperactivity, and loss of control of emotional responses. Thus, lesions in this area as a result of brain injury or dementia might lead to the inability to stop walking once one started or the inability to start walking or to do anything without a push. Likewise, on a psychological test such as the Bender-Gestalt, in which a person must copy a picture of dots, the person may be unable to stop doing so once she begins and so draw dots across her entire page and then onto and across the therapist's desk.

The parietal lobe is posterior to the Rolandic fissure. Areas 1 and 3 are called the primary sensory area. This area receives somatic-sensory information, especially information from touching things and sensations regarding bodily position. Lesions result in contralateral somatosensory impairment. Areas 5 and 7 are called the secondary sensory association area and are posterior to the primary sensory area. The secondary association area synthesizes (puts together) and elaborates somatosensory impulses, thereby permitting complex somatosensory perceptions such as stereognosis, the capacity to recognize objects by touch alone. Area 7 plays a role in the discrimination of somatosensory and visual signals. It is involved in body image and body recognition (which together are called *somatognosis*). Lesions of Area 5 result in astereognosis; lesions of Area 7 result in astereognosis, contralateral sensory impairment, or both.

Visual, auditory, and somatic stimuli are integrated in Areas 39 and 40. Thus, body schema (a sense of your arms and legs and height, the knowledge that your body parts belong to you, as well as knowing what your arm is) are "put together" here. Lesions result in asomatognosis, alexia, anomia, right-left disorientation, finger agnosia, or any combination of these. For example, in the delightful book, *The Man Who Mistook His Wife for a Hat,* neurologist Oliver Sacks presents the case of a man with severe asomatognosis. In a chapter titled, "The Man Who Fell Out of Bed," the patient did not recognize his leg as his own as a result of a brain lesion and, instead, believed it to be a severed leg in his bed. He persisted in trying to throw the horrible, severed, alien leg out of his bed and could not understand how or why he fell out of bed with it. This book by Sacks, as well as his many other books presenting neurological case studies (e.g., *Awakenings* became a popular movie starring Robin Williams as Sacks), are recommended as further readings that clarify brain-body relationships. Sacks's books are written much like novels, without technical jargon, and are highly informative.

The occipital lobe is at the posterior tip of the brain. Area 17 is the primary visual receptive area, with the left and right sides of it receiving visual information from the ipsilateral half of each retina. What you see is represented here, so in a neurological sense, your eyes are in the back of your head. Area 18 is the visual parareceptive area, immediately adjacent to Area 17. Visual images are integrated in Area 17, allowing us to recognize the things we see as what they are (e.g., to look at a dog and realize "That's a dog"); visual memories are stored in this area. Lesions and disturbances here therefore result in visual agnosia, but Area 19 must also be disturbed for that to happen. Area 19 is called the preoccipital area. This area integrates the functions of Areas 17 and 18 with the rest of the cortex. It controls visual recall, association, recognition, and orientation. Lesions and disturbances here result in visual illusions and hallucinations, disturbed spatial orientation and visual discrimination, and visual agnosia. A wonderful, sensitive example of a patient with lesions in this area (and other areas) and severe visual agnosia is also given in *The Man Who Mistook His Wife for a Hat,* by Oliver Sacks. The title refers to the sad fact that this patient's visual agnosia was so extreme that when asked to point to his hat, he pointed to his wife.

The temporal lobe is probably the single most important, and undoubtedly the single most complex, area of the brain. It is below and behind the Sylvian fissure. Areas 41 and 42 constitute the auditory receptive area and include the transverse temporal gyrus (called Heschl's area). Auditory impulses (what you hear) are represented here. *Lesions or seizures in this area can result in auditory illusions and hallucinations.* Areas 22 and 42 make up the auditory association area. If auditory memories are stored anywhere, they are stored in these two areas. Memory for patterns of sounds is believed to be stored here, and auditory stimuli are interpreted and understood as words or music here. Lesions in this area in the left hemisphere result in receptive aphasia, agraphia, and alexia. Lesions in this area on the right side of the brain result in inability to comprehend paralinguistics (tones of voice, inflections).

Area 43 is the gustatory area; what you taste (e.g., knowing that something tastes sweet or salty, recognizing the flavor of coconut) is represented here. Areas 28 and 35 together are the olfactory area; what you smell (e.g., the ability to smell coffee and recognize that smell) is represented here.

Finally, the temporal lobe is connected to the limbic system (which controls emotion) and to the hippocampus (which controls memory) as well. Thus, *the temporal lobe controls language, taste, smell, hearing, memory, and emotion.* Lesions or seizures in it result in everything from emotional changes (depression, anger, anxiety) to periods of lost time (engaging in actions with no memory for them) to aphasia and other language disturbances to auditory hallucinations.

Some Important Subcortical Structures

The *thalamus* receives impulses from the body and face and sends that information to the parietal cortex. The *hypothalamus* controls visceral functions—that is, temperature stability, appetite, sexual activity, sleep cycle, and so on, and through the pituitary, it controls the entire endocrine system. Hypothalamic lesions result in visceral symptoms.

The *basal ganglia* refers to the caudate, putamen, and globus pallidus. These structures, together with two others (the red nucleus and the substantia nigra), modify impulses from the motor cortex and so elaborate, integrate, and permit highly complex, voluntary motor activity. *Parkinson's disease* is a well-known neurological disorder involving a disturbance in these structures (specifically, in the substantia nigra). It is characterized by a diversity of highly complex, involuntary movements, including continual and severe muscular tremors (consisting of 4-8 movements per minute) of the hands, neck, and face; difficulty with swallowing, chewing, and speaking; disturbances in balance; akinesia, the inability to initiate movements; masklike facial expression; stiff gait, characterized by the upper body's moving forward ahead of the legs (as if the person has a board tied to his or her back and is being pulled forward by the head against his or her will); and a prototypical "pill-rolling" tremor (in which the hand moves involuntarily in a manner suggesting the constant rolling of a pill between the fingers). This progressive, degenerative neurological disorder is the result of the depletion of the neurotransmitter dopamine (because of atherosclerosis, encephalitis, and other diseases) from the substantia nigra, which is by and large destroyed. More than 1.5 million Americans suffer from Parkinson's disease (Dooneief et al., 1992; Stang, 1970), and the disease is accompanied by severe depression in 90% of those cases (see references). Although Parkinson's disease is a physical disorder with some psychiatric symptoms, we devote only this cursory attention to it because its major, prototypical symptoms are motoric (not psychological) and thus it is not misdiagnosed as a psychiatric disorder. Parkinson's disease is presented as an example of how disruption of a tiny brain structure or area can be manifested in severe neurological and psychological symptoms.

The subcortical structures that constitute the basal ganglia, along with the red nucleus, substantia nigra, and the nerve tracts that descend from the brain to the spinal motor neurons, together are sometimes called the *extrapyramidal nervous system*. Chronic use of antipsychotic (phenothiazine) drugs (e.g., Thorazine, Haldol, Mellaril) causes depletion of dopamine in the basil ganglia and related structures and results in drug-induced, severe Parkinson's-like neurological disorders called *extrapyramidal syndromes*. In addition to a pill-rolling tremor and the muscular rigidity and gait seen in Parkinson's, extrapyramidal syndromes entail other abnormal, involuntary movements, such as dystonia, arching of the back and a twisted posture, and akathesia, often manifested in constant pacing, chewing, and fidgeting. These extrapyramidal syndromes are caused solely by the use of antipsychotic drugs and are seen all too often among chronic mental patients diagnosed (correctly or incorrectly) as schizophrenic. One of these extrapyramidal syndromes, *tardive dyskinesia*, is irreversible: taking additional medications to restore dopamine functioning, or reducing the dosage of antipsychotics, or taking the patient off of the antipsychotics altogether does not halt the symptoms, which remain for the rest of the patient's life. In addition to all of the extrapyramidal and Parkinson's symptoms detailed above, tardive dyskinesia includes other bizarre, uncomfortable, involuntary movements, such as constant chin wagging, lip smacking and sucking movements, and the repeated, sudden protruding and retracting of the tongue (called "fly-catcher's tongue"). This irreversible, neurological disorder appears in 10% to 20% of patients who have been maintained on phenothiazines for an extended period of time (see Kane et al., 1986). Thus, efforts are made to treat those diagnosed as schizophrenic with the lowest possible dose of antipsychotics, and "drug holidays" (during which the patient does not take the antipsychotic drug) are also used to prevent extrapyramidal syndromes, tardive dyskinesia in particular (e.g., see Thaker et al., 1987).

The *limbic system* refers to the cingulate gyrus, the hippocampal gyrus, and all functionally associated nuclei—the amygdala, septal nuclei, nuclei of the hypothalamus, and portions of the basil ganglia. This system is the physical substrate of all emotion and is connected to the temporal lobes.

Finally, proprioceptive (information from sensory end organs) and vestibular (balance) impulses are represented in the cerebellum. Lesions result in disruption of balance, equilibrium, orientation in space, and posture.

Summary

Although far from complete, this cursory introduction to localization of function will facilitate understanding of why specific behavioral and other symptoms result from seizures localized to specific brain areas. As such, it can assist therapists not only in understanding a patient's symptoms but also in helping patients understand those symptoms. It is to the reader's advantage to become familiar with the names of various brain structures and with the basic nature of localization of function because such knowledge will facilitate interaction with medical specialists as well as understanding of their reports; definitions of the medical terms used are given in the glossary.

Likewise, it is particularly important to memorize the meaning of the various medical prefixes (e.g., *ipsi, contra, hemi, a, somata, stereo*) and suffixes (e.g., *kinesia, taxia, lexia, gnosia, graphia*) used in this chapter and to begin practicing using these terms to facilitate communication with medical specialists who tend to use such language and often have little time or desire to explain such terminology to a patient—let alone to that patient's therapist. In the final analysis, this kind of language is the *lingua franca* of medicine, the language through which medical professionals think and work, and the only language that they understand and respect, such that its use can be crucial to acquiring their assistance in providing the best services for women. For example, neurologists will pay more attention to a therapist who reports that her "patient" exhibits "bilateral ataxia and weakness after a hot bath," than to a therapist who reports that her "client" complains that she "feels weak and like she's lost all control of her body after a hot bath." The latter communication does not differ from what the patient herself would report and so would lead neurologists to wonder why they should "waste time" talking to a therapist who adds no information or understanding to the patient's report. In addition, the former communication is likely to be heard as "possible multiple sclerosis" (among other disorders) and the latter as "obvious somatization" in a woman psychotherapy patient (whose therapist may have failed to recognize it); only the therapist who communicates in the *lingua franca* of medicine will acquire the medical tests needed to help the woman being seen in therapy. This is to say that acquiring medical tests and other types of medical assistance for women in psychotherapy, by and large, is contingent on how the therapist communicates with medical professionals, which in turn is largely a function of the use of the *lingua franca* of medicine; that language (presented throughout this book and detailed in the glossary) must become part of the communication skills of the therapist. We address these issues in detail in the section on Clinical Practice Considerations.

With this cursory introduction to localization of function in hand, we can now turn to an examination of the symptoms that result from seizures in these various brain areas.

References

Dooneief, G., Miarabello, E., Bell, K., Marder, K., Stern, Y., & Mayeux, L. (1992). An estimate of the incidence of depression in Parkinson's disease. *Archives of Neurology, 49*, 305-307.

Kane, J. M., Woerner, M., Weinhold, P., et al. (1986). Incidence of tardive dyskinesia: Five-year data from a prospective study. *Psychopharmacology Bulletin, 20*, 387-389.

Sacks, O. (1985). *The man who mistook his wife for a hat and other clinical tales.* New York: Summit.

Stang, R. R. (1970). The etiology of Parkinson's disease. *Diseases of the Nervous System, 31*, 381-390.

Thaker, G. K., Tamminga, C. A., Alphs, L. D., et al. (1987). Brain γ-aminobutyric acid abnormality in tardive dyskinesia. *Archives of General Psychiatry, 44*, 522-531.

Generalized and Simple Focal Seizures

As discussed in Chapter 4, "Introduction to Seizure Disorders," seizures are categorized into two broad clusters called *generalized* (involving the entire brain) and *focal* (or partial, involving a small part of the brain) disorders. In this chapter, we provide a brief overview of the various types of generalized seizure disorders, followed by a similarly brief overview of the many types of focal seizure disorders. The focal seizure disorders discussed in this chapter are those with simple (or elementary) symptoms; those with more complex symptoms are detailed in Chapter 7. This discussion of generalized and simple focal seizure disorders is brief because these disorders can be, but are unlikely to be, misdiagnosed as psychiatric. Complex partial (focal) seizure disorder (CPS or temporal lobe epilepsy), on the other hand, is highly likely to be misdiagnosed as a variety of psychiatric disorders (e.g., as indicated by the case of Kate presented in the Introduction) and so is treated in detail in the next chapter.

Types of Generalized Seizures

Petit Mal Seizures

The most common of the generalized seizures are *petit mal* and *grand mal*. Petit mal seizures occur primarily in children. This type of seizure consists of simple "absence" attacks that last 5 or 10 seconds. These attacks are called absence attacks because during them the child appears to be (and in many ways is) "absent" from his or her activities. Typically, the child will suddenly stop whatever he or she is doing, stare blankly, and fail to respond to the environment; these behaviors indicate that a decrease in level of consciousness has occurred and that the child therefore is not aware of self or environment. The staring tends to involve an upward deviation of the eyes and some mild twitching of the eyes, eyelids, face, or extremities. Sometimes the absence is more complex and longer and in that case involves oral automatisms. The term *automatism* refers to any well-learned, simple, harmless behavior that is engaged in repeatedly and without conscious awareness during a seizure. Oral automatisms seen in absence attacks include repetitive lip smacking, chewing, and other mouthing movements. Flushing of the face and urinary incontinence may also be present. Petit mal tends to be associated with a bilateral, 3 cycles per second (cps) electroencephalogram (EEG) pattern. This disorder is typically benign and tends to end in adolescence.

People who experience petit mal seizures are generally otherwise normal neurologically and psychologically. Petit mal attacks in children, however, can be mistaken for psychological or behavioral problems and, in particular, may be mislabeled as disobedience or lack of attention by parents and school teachers. It is not a psychological or behavioral problem but instead a common seizure disorder easily diagnosed by EEG and controlled with seizure (anticonvulsant) medication.

One subtype of petit mal has a different EEG pattern (called a constant slow spike and wave). This type of petit mal is characterized by absence attacks, mental retardation, and underlying brain dysfunction. It is called *Lennox-Gastaut syndrome,* occurs in children, and has only a slight possibility of being misdiagnosed as psychopathology.

Grand Mal Seizures

Grand mal seizures are the most severe type of seizures. This type of seizure begins with an abrupt loss of consciousness, stiffening of the body (called the *tonic phase*), and an epileptic cry—a sound caused by the involuntary, forced expiration of air from the lungs through closed vocal cords. In the tonic phase there is also dilation of the pupils, biting of the tongue, and bladder and fecal incontinence. This tonic phase is followed by a brief period of trembling of the body lasting several seconds. This is followed by the *clonic phase.* The clonic phase consists of generalized, bilateral, severe jerks (convulsions) of the body and the limbs. These clonic movements gradually slow and cease. They are followed by a postictal stupor during which the patient is limp and unresponsive. The ictal (seizure) period lasts only 1 to 2 minutes, and the postictal (after seizure) state lasts 5 to 10 minutes. After the postictal period, the patient is awake but confused. If left undisturbed, he or she will sleep for several hours and awake with a headache and aching muscles.

Grand mal seizures may occur in people of any age. Typically, the person remains psychologically normal. This type of seizure disorder tends to be accurately diagnosed and is what most people have in mind when they think of epilepsy.

Myoclonic Seizures

Myoclonic seizures consist of brief, bilateral, involuntary jerks of the extremities, face, and body. Myoclonic seizures are not a specific entity and can occur as a symptom of many disorders, such as encephalitis, metabolic disorders, and degenerative disorders. Myoclonic seizures can occur at any age but are most often seen in children. Similarly, *tonic seizures* consist of brief stiffening and extension of the limbs and are associated with a fast-pattern EEG. These are seen most often in children with the Lennox-Gastaut syndrome. Likewise, *clonic seizures* involve jerking movements of the limbs and facial muscles and are also seen in children with the Lennox-Gastaut syndrome. All three of these types of seizures have the potential to be misdiagnosed as movement disorders, tics, or psychopathology. *Atonic and akinetic seizures* are brief and consist of suddenly falling to the ground. Both are seen in children with Lennox-Gastaut syndrome. Finally, *infantile seizures* entail tonic-like movements with the arms flung forward or outward. These episodes last a mere 1 to 4 seconds. These are seen in children (infants through age 4) and result from brain injury occurring at birth or in early childhood.

Types of Simple Partial or Focal Seizures

Partial or focal seizures are those that occur in only a small, focused (hence, focal) part (hence, partial) of the brain. Their symptoms depend on their specific localization. On the basis of symptoms, partial seizures can be divided into two types, those with elementary (simple) symptoms and those with more complex symptoms; only the former are addressed below.

Partial Seizures With Elementary Motor Symptoms

There are three types of partial seizures with elementary (simple) motoric symptoms. *Focal motor seizures* arise in the frontal cortex and involve tonic-clonic movements on the opposite side (contralateral) of the body. The movements often occur in a march (called a Jacksonian march). Jerking begins in the face and then progresses to include other areas of the body in an orderly sequence that reflects the representation of the body in the contralateral cortex. It is brief and often associated with postictal weakness that can last from 1 minute to 24 hours. *Adversive seizures* arise in the premotor area of the frontal lobe and are characterized by a deviation of the head, eyes, and body to the opposite side of the seizure focus. *Postural seizures* entail a tonic posturing of a part of the body. In one prototypical type, there is an elevation and posturing of the arm in a fencer's posture, with a deviation of the head and eyes toward the arm (as if the patient is looking at his or her hand). In this case, the seizure arises in the supplementary motor area between the frontal area and the precentral gyrus on the brain side opposite the elevated arm.

Partial Seizures With Elementary Sensory Symptoms

Any of the primary sensory areas can generate focal sensory seizures, but on the whole, there are four types of partial seizures with simple, sensory symptoms. *Somatic sensory seizures* originate in the sensory strip (or postcentral gyrus) of the parietal lobe and consist of tingling sensations and pins and needles sensations in a part of the body contralateral to the discharging focus. They can occur in any area or in a march (a tingling march) analogous to a Jacksonian march. These seizures can be misdiagnosed as signs of an anxiety disorder (particularly if the individual experiencing them interprets and reports them to clinicians as tension and anxiety) or as evidence of somatization. *Visual sensory seizures* occur with a seizure discharge in the occipital lobe and are characterized by unformed visual hallucinations, such as flashing lights or colors, or dimming of vision in the contralateral visual field. These can be misdiagnosed as an eye disorder, symptoms of migraine headache, or hysteria. *Auditory sensory seizures* occur when the focus is the superior temporal gyrus and consist of buzzing, ringing, and hissing sounds. These are either dismissed by the person who experiences them or misinterpreted as signs of anxiety, fatigue, or hysteria. Last, *vertiginous* (whirling-spinning) sensory seizures also arise from the superior temporal gyrus. These seizures can be nauseating. When interpreted as nausea and dizziness by the patient, these seizures can be readily misdiagnosed as hysteria or somatization.

Misdiagnosis of Partial Seizures
With Elementary Sensory Symptoms

Given the nature of their symptoms, it is clear that on the whole and for the most part, partial seizures with elementary sensory symptoms can be, but are unlikely to be, misdiagnosed as psychopathology. Our clinical experience indicates, however, that there is one circumstance in which these highly specific, simple epileptic symptoms are *likely* to be misdiagnosed as psychopathology—namely, when the person experiencing them attributes them to an esoteric or bizarre cause in a desperate effort to explain these symptoms to himself or herself and make sense of them. In our experience, *what clinicians often mistakenly identify as psychopathology (specifically, as paranoia) is not a physical symptom per se but the individual's causal attribution for that symptom,* an attribution whose bizarreness looms in the foreground of clinical attention like a red flag and so obscures the initial physical symptom, which subsequently is overlooked or forgotten. We believe that this process of patient misattribution-clinician misdiagnosis is an extremely common one and so illustrate it with the case of Jackie, as follows, and then provide some empirical evidence on the topic as well.

A Case Example: Jackie

Jackie was a 39-year-old, married White woman being seen as an outpatient at a large, community mental health center. She had been diagnosed as schizophrenic at the age of 25 and had received 14 years of therapy as well as a low dose of antipsychotics prior to one of the author's being called in for consultation on her case. The initial presenting symptom that had led to the diagnosis of schizophrenia 14 years prior was her delusion that the ghost or spirit of her dead mother was standing behind her, pushing her forward, spinning her around, occasionally slamming her face into the floor, and shocking her with electricity. Jackie had persisted in this delusion for 14 years, despite individual, group, couples, and drug therapy; she not only had shown no improvement at all in that time but now had several new delusions, including the claim that the winged insects nesting in her stomach would soon fly from her mouth and into the faces of the clinic staff. Hence, the consultation.

A brief history of Jackie's symptoms is provided here. This history was discovered by reading the original file on her. After 14 years at the mental health center, Jackie had dozens of files, each hundreds of pages long; the oldest of these (and the most important because it explained how her symptoms came about) were stored in a basement and forgotten—and so (unfortunately) never read—by contemporary clinic staff.

Since approximately age 20, Jackie repeatedly experienced the sensations of being spun around and pushed from behind, along with the occasional sensation of being dropped from a great height, of "the floor rushing up to my face and dropping down again." These sensations occurred several times during the day and often made her nauseous, so she treated her symptoms with over-the-counter drugs for nausea and dizziness. At night, while asleep, however, she had the additional sensation of whirling through space and of being electrocuted; these sensations were accompanied by a high-pitched buzzing sound and an inability to move—to rise, to call out to her husband about the experience. Although she found the nighttime sensations frightening, she ignored them because they were less frequent than the daytime ones and because they passed quickly, lasting less than a minute each time. The daytime sensations were disturbing to her, however, because of the nausea associated with them and because of their frequency and increasing intensity.

Specifically, as the frequency (10-20 per day) and intensity of her daytime sensations increased over the next 5 years, Jackie's behavior became odd. Now, when she had the sensation of being shoved from behind (as if a hand pushed on the back of her head) she literally flew forward in a manner consistent with being shoved. Likewise, when she had the sensation of spinning (as if someone behind her grabbed her arm and twirled her about), she would rock on her feet with unsteadiness and dizziness. Similarly, when she experienced the sensation of being dropped from a great height and watching the floor rush up to meet her nose, she would jerk her body back in a manner suggesting that she'd been running and then had screeched to a halt at the edge of a cliff. These sudden movements were noticeable and strange and drew increasing attention from her coworkers and husband. Her husband, in particular, was concerned that Jackie was acting strangely; it was one thing to complain of weird sensations and quite another to constantly and suddenly pitch forward, slamming into people and dropping things, when there was no one behind her. Jackie agreed that these sensations and experiences were abnormal but could not imagine what was wrong with her. Neither she nor her husband thought that she had a mental illness (she never said anything "crazy"), and they couldn't imagine a physical illness that would entail these symptoms. Thus, Jackie did not seek help from a physician; likewise, she did not come to the attention of mental health professionals—not until she finally found a way to explain these symptoms to herself.

Two years before the onset of these symptoms (when Jackie was about age 18), her mother had died (the manner was not specified in Jackie's old files). Jackie had a close relationship with her mother, whom she considered her source of inspiration and courage. Her mother had always stood behind her, offering support and encouraging her to struggle to be more than the "poor White trash" the family considered themselves to be. Her mother had constantly pushed Jackie to stay in high school and earn a diploma, to avoid getting pregnant young as she had done, and after finishing high school, to seek additional education that would allow her to get a job as a secretary or a nurses' aide. Her mother had pushed her to "make something" of herself, to acquire a job in a hospital or an office, to never become a high school dropout and a factory worker like her parents.

Jackie's mother died before Jackie finished high school. Jackie was depressed after her mother's death (though, apparently, not clinically so), particularly because her mother had never lived to see her graduate from high school, a goal Jackie met more to please her mother than herself. After a period of normal grief, Jackie continued along the lines that her mother had desired by taking a secretarial course, getting a job in an office as a file clerk, marrying a man who was a hardworking mechanic and earned a "decent" living, and slowly investigating other and "better" career options for herself. Soon, however, Jackie's heart was no longer in this struggle to improve herself; she no longer had the drive she'd had when her mother was alive, standing behind her, encouraging her, pushing her. Working as a file clerk was fine with her. Thus, Jackie devoted less and less energy to researching other careers and to furthering her education and finally ceased this altogether, satisfied to be a file clerk in an office, married to a hardworking man. She and her husband were not what her mother had hoped, but they were a step above poor White trash, and had both graduated from high school. Jackie decided that this was good enough. A few weeks later, her sensations and symptoms began.

After 5 years of her symptoms (by age 25), Jackie's and her husband's need to explain them was pressing. Jackie spent a lot of time thinking about her symptoms and discussing them with her friends, and one day, suddenly, the reason for these symptoms came to her in a flash of insight that made her feel calm and happy: It was the spirit, the ghost, of her mother, that caused these sensations. Her mother was standing behind her and pushing her to become something more. It was the spirit of her mother, smacking her on the back of the head as she had done many times in life, reminding Jackie to be more, to desire more. It was the spirit of her mother, spinning her around, demanding that she "take a hard look" at where she had been and then at how much farther she had to go. It was her mother slamming her face into the floor to teach her a lesson, coming to her during sleep and "shocking" her to help her "wake up" to the purpose of her life; it was her mother making her feel nauseous and sick about the life she had. It had to be her mother—that's why the sensations began when Jackie had "settled" for her current life. This was obvious.

Jackie revealed these insights to her husband. His response was that Jackie had finally lost her mind and needed help; pitching forward and slamming into people was weird, but claiming that her dead mother was the cause of that was just plain crazy. Thus, Jackie came to the attention of the mental health center where she was diagnosed as schizophrenic; her explanation for her symptoms became the focus of clinical attention and was interpreted as a paranoid delusion. Fourteen years prior to this, the staff had heard her entire history and so knew that Jackie's physical symptoms preceded her "delusion" by many years and that the latter was simply Jackie's theory about those symptoms. Unfortunately, they failed to recognize the significance of that; they failed to recognize her physical symptoms as a sign of a partial seizure disorder (localized to the superior temporal gyrus) with elementary, sensory (vertiginous and auditory) symptoms, so they dismissed those symptoms and subsequently labeled the very good explanation (in the context of her life) that Jackie had found for those symptoms as a mere delusion. Consequently, within 1 year of being seen at the mental health center, Jackie's new file no longer even mentioned the physical symptoms that were the genesis of her problems and referred only to her "delusion"; the delusion was now utterly incomprehensible in the absence of the physical symptoms it was meant to explain and thus necessarily "psychotic." This aspect of Jackie's case reveals what we regard as a sad truism of life—namely, that when a case of any type (psychiatric, child welfare, or legal) has been seen for many years and so passed from professional to professional, important details are slowly lost between the cracks of interpretations and lack of thoroughness; the loss of these details reduces and simplifies the person in question and inevitably renders him or her a monstrosity.[1] God (as Einstein once said) is in the details—the genesis of the problem and key to its comprehension are given in the details. No one at the mental health center who was currently involved in Jackie's case had ever read her original files containing the details on her physical symptoms; clearly, it is imperative for therapists to do so.

For the first 3 years of being seen at the clinic, Jackie's family history remained salient for the clinic staff; her relationship with her mother (but not her physical symptoms) was summarized and repeated in her new files and viewed as etiologically significant. Thus, for those years, her therapy had focused on her unexpressed hatred of her mother for pushing her so hard and her subsequent ambivalence regarding her mother's death. Jackie denied anger at her mother and denied ever wishing that her mother would die, but therapists insisted that this was there and called Jackie's claims "denial" and "resistance." This therapy, in conjunction with drug therapy, did not reduce the frequency of Jackie's symptoms, however. Thus, a few years later, Jackie's files no longer mentioned her initial physical symptoms nor even her relationship with her mother. The manufacture of a monstrosity was complete.

At the time of consultation, Jackie's (current) file indicated that she had persisted in her delusion for the past 14 years. Many years of individual, group, marital, and vocational therapy, in conjunction with 14 years of antipsychotic medication (which had elicited an extrapyramidal syndrome but not, thankfully, tardive dyskinesia) had not reduced any of her symptoms at all. The reason for consultation was that Jackie not only had failed to show any improvement in 14 years of treatment but also was now significantly worse. Along with her original sensations of being pushed and twirled by day and electrocuted by night, Jackie had several new sensations and complaints: her mother now was punching her in the stomach; ants were crawling around under her skin; her stomach was moving about inside her body and attempting to exit via her mouth; and winged insects were crawling around in her stomach and would one day, to the surprise of the entire cynical clinic staff, fly from her mouth when she opened it to answer their questions.

To resolve this case, the neurological nature of Jackie's original symptoms was explained to the clinic staff, and her original file used to demonstrate that her ostensible delusion was merely her attempt to make sense of what had been happening to her. The clinic staff happily agreed with this new interpretation because the details in her original file constituted irrefutable evidence, because the new view made sense of her absence of any other symptoms of schizophrenia (hallucinations, thought disorder, disturbance of affect, etc.), and because they, after all, were *not* the ones who had delivered the misdiagnosis.[2]

Likewise, Jackie's new delusions were explained as descriptions of new sensations, these being evidence of increases in the frequency of her seizures and in the size of the area of their discharge (i.e., spreading), this due to the failure to treat her seizures and to the use of antipsychotic drugs, which themselves are known to elicit seizures. The interdisciplinary team (a psychiatrist, two social workers, several psychiatric nurses, and assistants) agreed to slowly wean Jackie from antipsychotics, obtain an EEG and a physical exam to rule out other physical disorders that might be involved in her sensations, switch her to a trial of anticonvulsants irrespective of the EEG findings, discuss the new interpretation of her symptoms with her and her husband, follow her for 3 months, and if all was well, discharge her from the mental health center.

A follow-up 4 months later with the clinic staff revealed that Jackie's EEG had been positive, no other physical disorders discovered, and her physical symptoms controlled by anticonvulsants. Unfortunately, after 14 years of believing that her dead mother was the cause of her sensations, Jackie still had trouble rejecting this belief (something social psychologists call "belief perseverance"); she understood and accepted that she had seizures but now suspected that perhaps her dead mother caused the seizures. Her husband, on the other hand, immediately accepted the new neurological conceptualization (because his wife's only "craziness" had been her explanation for her seizures) and threatened to sue the mental health center for robbing Jackie of "the best 14 years" of her life by "making her believe she was nuts when she weren't crazy at all." He was equally angry about the additional symptoms that Jackie still displayed (e.g., sensitivity to sunlight, breast lactation) as a result of 14 years of antipsychotic medications.

Jackie's case is presented as a (sad) example of one of the many processes through which a physical disorder is misdiagnosed as psychiatric—namely, those cases in which the patient's explanation for (attribution regarding) his or her physical symptoms is itself regarded as a symptom of paranoia and the original physical symptoms subsequently forgotten. Because we believe that this process is a common one and accounts for many cases of ostensible paranoid disorders, we present other similar cases in the next chapter and discuss some empirical evidence on this process in what follows.

Empirical Evidence for the Patient Misattribution-Clinician Misdiagnosis of Paranoia Process

The notion that a person's attribution for a physical symptom can appear to be a paranoid delusion, become the focus of clinical attention, and then lead to a psychiatric misdiagnosis stems not only from our clinical experience but also from empirical evidence. For example, Zimbardo, Andersen, and Kabat (1981) attempted to unravel the well-known relationship between hearing loss in old age and the prevalence of paranoia among the elderly, a correlation first noted by Emil Kraepelin more than a century ago. Zimbardo and his colleagues hypothesized that when the elderly slowly lose their hearing they experience this (obviously) as not quite being able to hear what others (family members in particular) are saying. Instead of attributing this to a loss of hearing (which they do not realize they have), the elderly misattribute this to whispering on the part of family members: Relatives standing a few meters away and talking among themselves are perceived as whispering together, and because the only reason to whisper is to exclude the elderly person from the discussion, the elderly person logically concludes that the whispering is about him or her. The elderly person then fills in the blanks—generates hypotheses about what his or her relatives are "whispering" about—and these projections inevitably consist of hostile, degrading comments and nefarious conspiracies and plots against them. This is followed by bizarre accusations and allegations from the elderly person, subsequent denials from the family, and further suspicions from the elderly person that inevitably end in that person's being (mis)diagnosed as paranoid.

To test this hypothesis, Zimbardo and his colleagues (1981) hypnotized a group of normal undergraduate students. All were given the suggestion that (when they saw the word *focus* on a screen) they would have trouble hearing. Half (the control group) were told that they would be aware of the fact that this was due to induced partial deafness, and half (the experimental group) were told nothing further. Thus, the control group was provided with an explanation for not being able to hear, and the experimental group (analogous to the elderly person) was given no explanation, and so would have to construct their own explanations for not being able to hear.[3] One at a time, a student from each group was sent to work with a small group of confederates (people who work for the researcher) on a simple task. The confederates did not know what the research was about and did not know which group (experimental or control) the subject belonged to; the confederates knew only that one student at a time would come to work with them, that they had been instructed by Zimbardo to laugh and joke among themselves *about the task* as soon as the word *focus* appeared on the screen, and that they would later be required to rate the behavior of the student who'd been sent to join them.

The results of this study were dramatic and fascinating: Students in the control group behaved normally during the cooperative task, were rated as such by the confederates, and scored normally on psychological tests. Students in the experimental group, on the other hand, became hostile, accusatory, and agitated (paranoid) because they experienced the confederates as whispering and because they believed (projected) that this whispering was about issues that were of great psychological concern to them (e.g., one student accused the confederates of whispering about his closet homosexuality). Students from the experimental group were rated as hostile and paranoid by confederates, and they scored as paranoid on psychological tests.

Thus, hearing loss can be misattributed by the patient to whispering on the part of relatives, which can result in the misdiagnosis of paranoia. Likewise, memory loss in old age, with a subsequent inability to recall where one has put things, can be misattributed by the patient to people stealing things—to being robbed—and again result in the misdiagnosis of paranoia. And as illustrated by Jackie's case, a diversity of odd, physical symptoms associated with seizures of the simplest type similarly can be imbued with an esoteric explanation or attribution and subsequently misdiagnosed as paranoid.

To avoid rendering this kind of misdiagnosis and to be sensitive to when it has occurred, therapists should be careful to take the following precautions:

- Read all files on patients, no matter how long these are.
- Pay attention to physical symptoms that preceded ostensible delusions and assess the extent to which delusions are the patient's theory about those symptoms.
- Insist on basic physical exams (hearing, EEG) and psychological tests (of memory functions and the presence of psychosis) for all patients.
- Strongly suspect that an organic disturbance is the case when the patient exhibits a paranoid delusion but simultaneously fails to exhibit the associated, prototypical symptoms of schizophrenia or psychosis in interview and on psychological tests.

We can turn now to an examination of partial seizures with complex symptoms.

Notes

1. By "monstrosity" we mean someone bizarre or horrible and utterly incomprehensible.

2. They had failed, they admitted, to read through 14 years of files on Jackie; that was problematic but (they said) something no one in a busy mental health center had time to do. It was not clear that the staff intended to change this aspect of their behavior—despite the finding that a second case (on which consultation was requested) was remarkably similar to Jackie's and in part again the result of failure to read old files.

3. This important experiment is briefly summarized here and was more complex than this summary suggests; the reader is referred to the Zimbardo et al. (1981) article for the details of the study.

Reference

Zimbardo, P. G., Andersen, S. M., & Kabat, L. G. (1981). Paranoia and deafness: An experimental investigation. Science, 212, 1529-1531.

Complex Partial Seizure Disorder

Temporal Lobe Epilepsy

In this chapter, we discuss the myriad of symptoms associated with temporal lobe epilepsy. Partial (focal) seizures with complex symptoms (called complex partial seizures [CPS], psychomotor, or temporal lobe epilepsy [TLE]) arise from the temporal lobe and involve the connected limbic system and several diencephalic structures as well. These seizures manifest themselves in personality, affective, cognitive, and behavioral changes. This type of seizure disorder is highly likely to be misdiagnosed as any number of psychiatric disorders and is presented in detail.

We can best understand complex partial seizure disorder by examining its symptoms in terms of the stages of this seizure disorder. Some have delineated the following as the primary stages of a complex partial seizure:

1. Prodromal stage
2. Ictal stage
   a. Primictal stage
   b. Ictal amnesic stage
3. Postictal stage
4. Interictal stage
5. Epileptic psychosis

Prodromal Stage and Its Symptoms

Many epileptic patients report changes in mood and affect that begin long before the onset of the seizure. Usually, this prodromal feeling persists for hours, but for many, it lasts for 3 to 7 days. The prodromal symptoms are vague feelings of being generally moody, depressed, anxious, or uptight. Many feel a low level of constant anger, irritation, or annoyance, accompanied by generalized unhappiness and malaise, and they get into constant arguments. This is coupled with an experience of decreased ability to concentrate. This portion of the seizure is readily misdiagnosed or dismissed as a mood disturbance. Unfortunately, because such seizures in women are often correlated with menstruation (where hormonal changes push the damaged, central nervous system over the brink, so to speak), this portion of the seizure is often misinterpreted as a so-called premenstrual syndrome. Typically, however, patients (women in particular) reporting these symptoms are misdiagnosed as depressed.

Ictal Stage and Its Symptoms

The ictal stage has several important features. First, although the symptoms of the ictal stage vary from patient to patient, each patient tends to exhibit precisely the same symptoms every time he or she has a seizure. Second, the ictal stage (the period of the seizure) is very brief and lasts about 60 to 90 seconds. During that 60 to 90 seconds, the patient engages in a highly stereotyped sequence of behaviors that occur with every seizure. The highly stereotyped and episodic nature of the symptoms at this stage can help us differentiate CPS from psychiatric disorders. Finally, the ictal stage can be divided into the portion that people remember (the aura or primictal phase) and the portion that they do not recall (the ictal amnesic phase). People often think of the primictal symptoms as a warning sign of a seizure to come; in fact, however, this aura or primictal event is the first stage of a seizure that already is under way. The primictal event that the patient remembers is not directly observable but is reported by the patient. The behaviors exhibited during the brief ictal amnesic period are observable but not recalled by the patient. This amnesia can persist beyond the seizure discharge and into the beginning of the postictal phase.

Primictal Stage and Its Symptoms

The prodromal phase is an hour or even a week of moody, anxious, irritability that precedes the actual seizure. We might think of it as the behavioral and psychological manifestation of a brain that is storing up abnormal electrical activity that will finally be relieved in a sudden abnormal discharge. Next, the seizure begins with any of a multitude of primictal or aura events; these are remembered by the patient and are always the same for each patient. The most common primictal events are described and categorized below.

Elementary Auditory Illusions

Illusions are misperceptions of actual environmental stimuli, whereas hallucinations are perceptions of nonexistent environmental stimuli. Elementary auditory illusions are misperceptions of actual sounds. Things are heard as louder than normal, softer than normal, or as increasing or decreasing in rhythm or tone. This often is reported to others in an effort to check if things sound that way to them, too. These specific auditory illusions indicate that CPS focus (the precise localization of the abnormal discharge) is probably the superior temporal gyrus, near the primary receptive area, in either hemisphere. Thus, after a week of being moody and argumentative, the person suddenly asks if things sound too loud or demands that the television, which she perceives as blaring, be turned down. This brief event is overlooked by everyone.

Elementary Auditory Hallucinations

These tend to be indistinct noises that the patient finds difficult to describe. People report hearing a murmur, a buzz, wind blowing, a whisper, a hum, trickling water, the ticking of a clock, footsteps, a closing door, clapping, a dish breaking, or shots of a machine gun. The common feature of all elementary auditory hallucinations is that patients recognize them as pathological in character. The patient hears something, attempts to locate the source of the sound, and failing to find it, regards the event as odd at best. Indeed, typically, people with psychologically generated hallucinations can describe them in great detail and see nothing odd about hallucinating, whereas people with organic hallucinations find it difficult to describe what they are hearing and are often disturbed by the event because they know that hallucinating is pathological.

Thus, after a week of being moody and argumentative, the person suddenly asks if others hear someone knocking at the door or if others heard the doorbell ring; again, this brief event is overlooked by everyone.

Complex Auditory Hallucinations

Musical Type. The person reports hearing a melody and usually reports hearing the same melody. Sometimes, people will report that they hear voices singing but are unable to distinguish the words. Also, sometimes, musical instruments or an orchestra are heard. The intensity of musical hallucinations varies; sometimes they are distant, sometimes closer, sometimes deafening.

Verbal Type. These auditory hallucinations may involve single words or complete sentences. Often, the hallucination consists of a voice giving orders or advice to the patient and is readily misdiagnosed as psychogenic. Other common verbal auditory hallucinations include hearing voices mumbling or a group of voices with the words being unclear. In most cases, in an effort to explain and understand these voices (which are regarded as pathological by the patient), the patient arrives at a theory about them; this theory can be difficult to distinguish from a delusion and increases the chances of a psychiatric misdiagnosis. Yet the patient nonetheless regards the voices, in all organic cases, as pathological—that is, as something people are not supposed to experience and as something therefore requiring a good explanation.

For the most part, affective, rather than content, features of the heard voices dominate the presentation. Whereas the schizophrenic is disturbed by *what* the voices are saying and can describe that well, the organic patient is disturbed by the *mood of the voices* and cannot describe what they are saying. The CPS patient reports that the voice(s) sound threatening, angry, mean, or sad, for example, and that is why they are disturbing.

Thus, after a week of being moody and argumentative, the person believes that he or she hears people mumbling and goes to see where the voices are coming from; this brief event is overlooked by everyone, or depending on what he or she hears, is interpreted as psychogenic in origin. A patient's response to such brief, primictal, verbal hallucinations can lead to a serious psychiatric diagnosis, however, as indicated in the case that follows.

A Case Example: Mindy

Several years ago, one of the authors was assigned a patient, Mindy, a 34-year-old, White, married woman; she was on an inpatient, acute psychiatric ward and had been diagnosed as having a severe, schizotypal personality disorder. Mindy's presenting symptoms were the delusion of being a medium for the dead and the hallucination of hearing the dead speak. On close questioning, it was revealed that the Mindy frequently heard voices mumbling—an entire group of sad, angry voices mumbling something that she could not understand. She searched for the source of these voices and, finding none, regarded hearing them as pathological. Over a period of months, she sought for an explanation of this pathological event and finally decided that the voices must be those of the dead and that she therefore must be a medium. Thus, she

Table 7.1   Organic Versus Psychiatric Delusions and Hallucinations

When verbal hallucinations and associated delusions are psychiatric in origin,
   The delusion precedes the hallucination,
   The voices of the hallucination are understandable and singular,
   The patient focuses on the *content* of the voices, and
   The patient does not sense anything odd about hallucinating.

When verbal hallucinations and associated delusions are organic in origin,
   The hallucination precedes the delusion,
   The delusion follows and is the patient's explanation for the hallucination,
   The voices of the hallucinations are not clear,
   There is typically more than one voice (usually a group).
   The mood of the voices is emphasized,
   The patient believes that hallucinating is a very odd event and a sign of a disorder, and
   The patient is normal in other respects; other "psychotic" symptoms are strangely absent.

regarded hallucinating as pathological and simultaneously attributed a highly esoteric meaning to the hallucinations in an effort to make sense of them. *Her ostensible delusion was her attempt to make sense of (causal attribution regarding) her primictal event,* something that is common in these cases, as detailed in the previous chapter. An electroencephalogram (EEG) with nasal leads found clear, left-lateralized temporal lobe epilepsy. She was switched from a low dose of an antipsychotic to an anticonvulsant medication and the voices disappeared in 24 hours. Her remaining difficulties for which counseling was needed involved her disappointment at the loss of her status as a medium, a status that raised her low self-esteem and made her neglectful husband pay attention to her.

In general, then, there are signs that can be used to differentiate psychiatric from organic delusions and hallucinations. These are summarized in Table 7.1.

In the preceding case, the diagnostic team (chief psychiatrist, medical residents, two psychologists on the admissions unit) did not feel comfortable in diagnosing Mindy as schizophrenic because she did not meet full criteria for the diagnosis. Hallucination and delusion aside, Mindy had shown no deterioration, no premorbid signs, no affective disturbance, or the like. Simultaneously, however, she was hallucinating, something one doesn't expect in personality disorders. Such inconsistent symptoms are often a reliable sign of a physical disorder. There are exceptions to this hallucination-delusion rule, however (e.g., the interictal psychosis of TLE), but generally, the above holds.

The Paliacousia Subtype of Verbal Hallucination.   One phenomenon related to these verbal hallucinations that appears in some patients is called *paliacousia.* In the course of a real conversation, the patient seizes on a word or words and then hears them over and over again, uncontrollably, in a hallucinatory fashion. The word or words are heard repetitively and intrude on other thoughts and concentration. This neurological condition is often misdiagnosed as an obsession or as a psychotic or prepsychotic symptom. Sometimes, such complex auditory verbal hallucinations precede or accompany aphasia; in some cases, aphasia is manifested only in such hallucinations. In these cases, patients complain of hearing incomprehensible words, distorted sentences, or a foreign language.

Studies of hallucinations have found that verbal hallucinations are the most common experience (followed by musical hallucinations) in neurological pathology (tumors or seizures) involving the temporal lobes. For two thirds of these patients, the voices were familiar—they "sound like" someone the patient knows or has known—and this increases the chances of misdiagnosing them as psychopathology. In terms of localization, these hallucinations appear to be associated with pathology in the area surrounding Heschl's gyri. As for hemispheric lateralization, most agree that auditory hallucinations can result from lesions or seizures in either hemisphere. Nonetheless, however, studies by Hecaen and Albert (1978a, 1978b) have found that the left hemisphere is more frequently involved in verbal auditory hallucinations.

Visual Illusions and Hallucinations

A second type of primictal event or aura is any variety of visual illusions and hallucinations. *Visual illusions and hallucinations always have an organic, rather than a functional or psychiatric, etiology.* Typically, these, as well as the elementary auditory illusions described previously, are manifestations of temporal lobe seizures due to epilepsy, brain tumors, or drug or alcohol abuse.

The term *visual illusion* refers to modifications of the visual perception of objects in terms of size, shape, movement, and the like. These illusions are usually *paroxysmal* (namely, they appear as a manifestation of epilepsy). Sometimes, however, they appear with migraine attacks without epilepsy. There are two major categories of visual illusions: *elementary illusions* and *complex illusions.*

Elementary Visual Illusions. These entail changes in the perceptual qualities of an object. Common illusions are (a) modification in the size of an object (e.g., macroscopia or microscopia), (b) modification of object size along a single dimension (objects look stretched or flat), (c) blurring of outlines of objects, (d) disappearance of the object's color or a uniform tint to all objects,

(e) illusion of movement of objects, and (f) illusion of increasing or decreasing pace of movement (people seem to be walking too fast or in slow motion).

Complex Visual Illusions. These entail perceived changes of three-dimensional visual space. The most common is the telescoping of objects (they seem small and far away). Such visual illusions are typically described by patients as "things look stretched," "like in a fun-house mirror." Such illusions tend to be associated with seizures in the right hemisphere's temporo-occipital region.

Olfactory and Gustatory Hallucinations

A third type of primictal event entails the fleeting perception of a strange taste or smell or bizarre sensations, such as the stomach rising. Or there is the sense of pressure from the stomach that rises to throat and causes a feeling of choking. This primictal event can readily be misinterpreted as somatization, hysteria, or globus hystericus. Some of these symptoms were seen in the case of Jackie, detailed in the previous chapter.

The "Dreamy State"

This type of aura was described by Hughlings Jackson (see Taylor, 1931) more than 100 years ago. It is a sudden, general change in perception. Usually, it takes the form of *déjà vu* (strange familiarity of the unfamiliar), *jamais vu* (strange unfamiliarity of the familiar), or depersonalization and derealization. Sudden feelings of fear, anxiety, or sadness are often associated with these primictal events. Whereas déjà vu and jamais vu are ordinarily dismissed by patient and clinician alike, sudden (i.e., paroxysmal) fear, anxiety, sadness, depersonalization, or derealization tend to be misdiagnosed as psychopathology.

Thus, after a week of being irritable and unhappy, the patient experiences and reports one of the preceding symptoms. These are so brief (i.e., a matter of seconds) each time they occur, that they are often ignored. In other cases, they are misdiagnosed as psychopathology. This is particularly likely to occur if the patient, experiencing this event once per month for 10 years, has generated an esoteric explanation for it.

Ictal Amnesic Stage and Its Manifestations

The next portion of the seizure consists of specific behaviors lasting only about 60 seconds for which the patient has amnesia. Although the primictal event is a private one that the clinician cannot observe, the behaviors of the ictal amnesic period are observable.

First, ongoing activity (such as talking) stops. This is followed by about 30 to 60 seconds of automatisms, of highly stereotyped, well-learned behaviors that are carried out automatically during the CPS while the patient is in an altered state of consciousness. Typical automatisms are unbuttoning the shirt, untying and retying the shoes, or brushing the hair. There are often also stereotyped, brief oral automatisms such as chewing or lip smacking. Scratching, stamping, or kicking is often seen. This ends quickly, and the patient enters the postictal stage.

Thus, after a week of being irritable and moody, the patient goes to the front door because she thought she heard the doorbell ring. She returns and tells her significant other that she heard the doorbell but no one was there. Her significant other indicates that he or she never heard anything. The patient then picks up a brush and begins to brush her hair or begins to chew. If her significant other does not speak to her for a few moments, no one will be aware of these symptoms or of the patient's absence (decreased level of consciousness). Thus, the prodromal, primictal, and ictal amnesic behaviors can be overlooked. Alternatively, as in the case of Mindy, after a week of being moody, the patient tells her husband that the voices of the dead are back. Then she begins to absently brush her hair while her husband (without her awareness) is asking her what the voices are saying. Her failure to answer, her specific primictal event, and her explanation for it, are misunderstood as psychopathology, and her husband talks her into being admitted to the local psychiatric hospital.

Postictal Stage Manifestations

The postictal period generally lasts 2 to 10 minutes, but in some it can persist for an hour. In this stage, relatively simple, repetitive, automatic acts appear. These are then followed by more complex automatisms, such as packing, unpacking, singing, undressing, showering, washing dishes, or shining shoes. These are usually *harmless routine activities* carried out for several minutes in a decreased state of consciousness (i.e., the patient isn't aware of what he or she is doing) while patients attempt to reorient themselves. If no one attempts to talk to the patient during this period, the entire event may be overlooked. Alternatively, if anyone was talking to the patient when she suddenly began to pack, wash dishes, or sing, the behavior will be misunderstood as psychopathology.

Although in most cases the postictal behavior is harmless, in some cases, complex and deviant behavior appears, including postictal violence (Blumer, 1976) with amnesia for it, as indicated in the example below.

A Case Example

A recent local television news story reported the case of a 17-year-old, African American boy's being arrested in a stereo store for attempted robbery. The boy had smashed the windows of the store with the trash cans from the sidewalk and then stepped inside. The police, alerted by the store alarm system, arrived and arrested him at the scene. What was odd about this from our perspective was that the boy hadn't stolen anything and hadn't tried to escape. Rather, when the police and news cameras arrived (which took quite some time), he was simply standing amid the broken glass, quite still, and appeared disoriented. When asked why he'd done this by a mindless reporter, the boy stared blankly and then said, "I don't know. I don't know. I guess I just wanted to." Although this could be interpreted as the typical affective blunting and indifference seen in psychopathy, we suspected that he had no memory of breaking the window and no idea of what he was doing standing in the store. Why hadn't he run when he heard the sirens? Why hadn't he taken anything? Why did he simply stand there as the cameras and reporters and police surrounded him? Was this an attempt to rob the store or a neurological symptom—postictal violence with amnesia?

In addition to postictal violence with amnesia, postictal hypersexuality with amnesia can also occur; this can range from being suddenly sexually excited to automatic orgasms and lasts 10 to 15 minutes (Blumer & Walker, 1967; Blumer, 1970, see References and Bibliography).

Interictal Stage Manifestations: The Temporal Lobe Epilepsy (TLE) "Personality"

In the interictal period (between seizures), patients with CPS exhibit a specific set of characteristics and behavioral propensities that seem much like a personality syndrome. Between seizures, this is what the patient is usually like as a person. The reason for this odd collection of characteristics is that, between clinical seizure periods, the EEG is not normal. Instead, there are some signs of persistent, subclinical seizure activity localized to the medial aspects of one or both temporal lobes. This chronic, excessive neuronal activity in the limbic system is assumed to be responsible for the reliable and specific set of traits seen in CPS patients. This interictal personality is often confused with a variety of personality disorders (e.g., borderline) as well as with affective disorders (e.g., depression). The interictal personality consists of 18 traits according to David Bear (1979a, 1979b; Bear & Fedio, 1977), Benson and Blumer (1975), and Blumer (1971, 1975, 1977), and these can be clustered into the three general personality factors that David Bear called *global hyposexuality, viscosity,* and *deepened emotionality.* The reader is referred to Bear (1979a, 1979b; Bear & Fedio, 1977), Benson and Blumer (1975), and Blumer (1971, 1975) for a more detailed description of this personality syndrome; the description of the TLE personality that follows relies solely on their research, whereas descriptions of other CPS symptoms are based on the numerous studies by the variety of authors listed in the Bibliography.

Global Hyposexuality

The patient has a chronic, global, absence of sexual desires and absence of an interest in sex and/or rarely experiences genital arousal. The patient with onset of CPS before puberty has never had an interest in sex and is not concerned by his or her hyposexuality. For patients with late-onset CPS, the hyposexuality is a matter of great concern because it represents a change. Many of these patients therefore experiment with a variety of sexual behaviors (usually homosexual ones) in an attempt to regain sexual feelings. Others engage in a variety of deviant sexual acts (usually transvestism, fetishism, and exhibitionism) in an effort to regain genital arousal. The woman presented in the Introduction, Kate, had late-onset CPS and so engaged in a variety of sexually deviant acts with the hope of achieving genital arousal.

Viscosity and Circumstantiality

This refers to the tendency to stick to, to adhere to, each thought, feeling, or activity. Patients proceed laboriously in their speech and clarify every detail. Their stream of conversation is excessive, tangential, and circumstantial as they follow loosely associated tangents, before finally coming back and finishing their original thought. They are overinclusive, giving excessive background details; precise times, dates, and places; cross-sectional and longitudinal perspectives on the facts while describing those facts; and a variety of circumstantial, nonessential details. A simple question is responded to with a long, circuitous discussion before the answer is given so that the therapist feels that this person simply cannot answer a simple question. The patients believe that nothing is trivial and so that nothing can be left out. Minor

issues, simple questions, and passing thoughts are given the time and emphasis of things important. In addition, every single detail is considered in terms
of its "rightness versus wrongness." This circumstantial, preseverative speech
looks schizotypal or borderline; it is most likely to be misdiagnosed as such
or as a sign of a subtle thought disorder. Kate, the woman described in the
Introduction, exhibited these symptoms and was misdiagnosed as having a
borderline personality disorder.

Related to this verbosity and viscosity is hyperethicality or hyperreligios-
ity. All issues, including minor ones, are reduced to or elevated to deciding
good versus bad or right versus wrong. There is an obsession with doing what
is right, fair, just, and good that can be mistaken for perfectionism or obsessive-compulsive ruminating. Some patients join extreme, esoteric religious
cults. Others change their religion or talk about religious issues incessantly.
These behaviors can be misdiagnosed as prepsychotic, obsessive-compulsive,
or manic. Kate exhibited these symptoms as well, and these were misunderstood as obsessive ruminating.

The combination of viscosity and hyperethicality often leads to *general
hypergraphia,* in which the patients keep countless notes, notebooks, logs,
and journals on absolutely everything and consider these scribblings important. Some write essays on moral topics. Most of all, they write long letters
and frequent notes to their physicians, therapists, ministers, congresspeople,
and the like. These notes and letters are hyperethical, circumstantial, overinclusive, and overdetailed; the writing matches the quality of the speech. This
behavior looks obsessive-compulsive or manic and can be readily misdiagnosed as such. *This hypergraphia is an important, differential diagnostic sign*
of temporal lobe epilepsy versus psychiatric disorder. Kate, as the reader may
recall, exhibited chronic hypergraphia.

Deepened Emotionality

The long-winded speech of temporal lobe epileptics tends to be full of
emotion, and this increased emotionality contributes to the viscosity. Emotions are intensified and felt deeper. The patient is also viscous about the
feeling or emotion and won't let it go. Every feeling, no matter how fleeting,
must be discussed, explored, and magnified. Issues of right or wrong are
central at all times. Patients are either highly good-natured, kind, helpful, and
hyperethical; moody and irritable; or fluctuate between these extremes. Others are dead serious, somber, and hyperethical but have explosive periods of
verbal aggression. Irrespective of which pattern the patient exhibits, almost
all also have periods of severe depression.

Mood disorders seen along with this personality syndrome depend on the age of the patient. In young adult CPS patients, there is a rapid cycling of mood, with shifts from depressed to hostile within hours. The younger the patient, the more extreme the episodes of anger are. In older adult patients, the mood swings involve severe depression with ruminations about being punished or deserving punishment. These patients often present depression and anxiety as their chronic mood, with periods of suicide attempts and periods of hostility and irritability. The depressed episode lasts for hours or days and is then followed by periods of brooding, ruminating, and anxious irritability with oversensitivity, and paranoid ideation. These mood swings often end in a seizure, and the affective cycle begins anew.

In other patients, it ought to be noted, there is a postictal psychosis that looks like schizophrenia or bipolar disorder. This period of florid psychosis lasts 12 to 24 hours. There may be paranoia, grandiosity, religiosity and sudden religious conversions, and auditory hallucinations. The underlying personality is CPS (deepened affect, viscous speech, hyperethicality) rather than schizoid, however. Thus, during the psychotic episodes, affect is neither flat, blunted, nor inappropriate; instead, affect is deepened and intense. For patients with frequent, severe CPS, an epileptic dementia can appear, characterized by the progressive deterioration of cognitive functions (e.g., attention span, memory, etc.).

In addition to the preceding personality syndrome, all CPS patients also tend to exhibit (a) paroxysms of explosive anger and, (b) if the seizures begin before puberty, *generalized hyperactivity* that can be readily misdiagnosed as an attention deficit disorder; it is associated with a paroxysmal rage that can lead the entire behavioral picture to be misdiagnosed as delinquency in young patients. Furthermore, in general, (c) *frankly psychotic episodes,* with the prototypical symptoms of schizophrenia or bipolar disorder, can and do appear in many patients under physical or emotional stress. These psychotic periods are exacerbations of the seizure disorder; they are symptoms related to and caused by CPS and are not schizophrenia or bipolar disorder per se. Treating the psychotic episodes as if they are psychogenic in origin by prescribing an antipsychotic or lithium exacerbates the symptoms such that the patient appears to be getting worse. Increasing the dosage of the antipsychotic in response to this ostensible "deterioration" further magnifies the symptoms and increases them while precipitating other symptoms as well. Thus, as in the case of treating the depressive symptoms seen in endocrinological disorders with antidepressants, likewise, treating the psychotic symptoms seen in CPS with antipsychotics only makes the symptoms worse because the patients, in either case, do not have psychiatric disorders.

Finally, some CPS patients develop what is called *poriomania*. During a prolonged ictal period, the patient wanders off and engages in ordinary, stereotyped activities without consciousness and later "wakes up" having lost time—hours, days, or even a month. *This looks like multiple personality and/or fugue* and can be readily misdiagnosed as such. It can be distinguished from those psychiatric disorders by the absence of a dynamic motivation (of discriminative stimuli) for the lost time and by the ordinariness of the behavior they are told they engaged in during the lost time.

A Case Example

In a highly publicized, television news case that occurred in California in December 1994, a 16-year-old African American girl with a history of brain damage and mental retardation was "captured" after "kidnapping" two small children that she had been asked to baby-sit. Many police officers had searched frantically for the missing children for several hours, and the distraught mother appeared on the news. The case was solved quickly when, to their surprise, the police found the kidnapper and the missing children in kidnapper's own home, where she had taken them (instead of watching them in their mother's home as agreed). After questioning, it was clear that the kidnapper had no memory of how she and the children had arrived at her apartment. When the police kicked in her door and awakened her (she was asleep), she was as surprised as the police were to find the children there, playing on the floor in her apartment and to find herself there asleep in her own bed. She said, "It's like a dream, you know? Like . . . they was . . . just here, somehow." When her history of brain pathology (unspecified) was revealed to the police and her failure to harm the children or demand a ransom highlighted (along with her lack of memory for any of the events), her "crime" was overlooked, and she was not charged. The officer in charge of the investigation of this case called it a "misunderstanding" of the behavior of someone with known brain damage and cognitive deficits.

This case, like the previous news case, probably represents temporal lobe seizures associated with underlying, generalized brain pathology; indeed, the symptom of lost time in the "kidnapping" case is the classic, well-documented CPS symptom poriomania. The possibility that the people in both news cases have temporal lobe pathology is increased by the fact that both of the ostensible criminals were lower-class African Americans. As such, in all probability, their mothers had poor prenatal and postnatal care; there were subsequent complications in their deliveries (e.g., low birth weight, anoxia); their early childhood nutrition was poor; and their childhood health care was poor (such that prolonged, high fevers could occur). These strong correlates and consequences of poverty are sufficient to cause diffuse brain damage and a seizure disorder.

Thus, we not only question how many ostensibly "mentally ill" people have misdiagnosed, treatable neurological and endocrinological disorders, we also question how many putative, young "criminals," "juvenile delinquents," and "gang bangers" represent misdiagnosed, treatable neurological disorders—particularly in light of studies that have found abnormal EEGs (Weiner et al., 1966) and abnormal scores on neuropsychological tests (Berman & Siegal, 1976) among delinquents. How much of the nation's crime, committed by poor, young people such as those described here, could be prevented by providing prenatal and postnatal care for the poor and nipping these neurological disorders in the bud? Could a national health care program prevent juvenile delinquency? It would cost the nation less to provide prenatal care for the poor and to provide neurological screening for all children when they enter elementary school in order to prevent and control neurological disorders than it costs our nation in lives, property, time, money, police, and lawyers to hunt, prosecute, and house delinquents and young criminals who in all likelihood have neurological disturbances (see Berman, 1972; Berman & Siegal, 1976). Although the violence and ostensible delinquency associated with specific types of temporal lobe seizures (e.g., the 14-and-6 positive spike seizure pattern) are not the focus of this book (because violence is rarely seen among women), some references on that topic are provided in the Bibliography at the end of the book for the interested reader.

Interim Summary

The typical CPS patient has been given the misdiagnosis of an affective disorder diagnosis on Axis I (bipolar, atypical depression, etc.) and borderline or some other personality disorder on Axis II. Others have been misdiagnosed as having hysteria, hypochondriasis, multiple personality disorder, or anxiety disorder or as having episodic dyscontrol syndrome. Although we know of no evidence indicating that CPS is more common among women than among men, *depression, anxiety disorders, multiple personality disorder, hysteria, and borderline personality are all symptoms that women exhibit significantly more often than do men* and are diagnoses that women receive significantly more often than do men (see references for the Introduction). It is highly likely that many of those women (41%-83% if we rely on the studies discussed in the Introduction) are misdiagnosed cases of CPS. CPS must be entertained as a possibility in all patients. A thorough psychosocial history that includes questions about birth weight and complications in delivery, mother's drug and alcohol use, and early childhood injuries and performance in school can assist in the accurate diagnosis of this disorder.

The Interictal Psychoses of TLE

That a chronic psychosis is associated with CPS has been known since the early 1900s. Research on the topic began with reports of cases of paranoid, hallucinated, deluded patients who had deteriorated to this state after many years of CPS. Typical of this research are the studies of Ounsted and Lindsay (1982). These researchers took a sample of 100 children who were diagnosed with CPS in 1964 by EEG results and then assessed them years later in 1977. The result was that 9 were diagnosed as schizophrenic. Although this may not seem to be a high percentage (9%), it is a rate of "schizophrenia" that is significantly higher than that of the general American population. In addition, this rate may be found to be much higher on later follow-ups because studies indicate that one must have CPS for 14 to 16 years for the interictal psychosis to develop.

Likewise, Slater and Beard (1963) examined 69 CPS cases and followed them for several years. Eleven exhibited psychotic confusional states, 46 exhibited the symptoms of paranoid schizophrenia, and 12 exhibited he-bephrenic symptoms. All 69 CPS cases exhibited psychosis despite their lack of the associated premorbid personality or family history that would predict schizophrenia. The psychosis started at age 29 to 30 years, after about 14 years of CPS and significantly later than the standard age of onset for schizophrenia (age 20). Perseveration of affect and hallucinations (auditory/visual) with religious and grandiose delusions were common in these patients.

In general then, researchers have found a fairly consistent relationship between CPS and a schizophrenia-like psychosis that emerges after and because of 14 or more years of untreated CPS. By the "schizophrenia-like psychosis" of CPS, researchers mean that, after being untreated for 14 to 18 years (not diagnosed correctly, not treated with anticonvulsants), CPS patients begin to exhibit auditory or visual hallucinations or both; systematized paranoid or grandiose delusions (with a marked religious flavor); ideas of influence; paranoid ideation; and thought disorder (circumstantiality and loose association) but all *in the presence of appropriate, warm but intense and deepened affect* (instead of the flat, blunted, or inappropriate affect seen in schizophrenia). Mystical delusions and ideation are common (and secondary to patients' attributions and explanations for their CPS primictal events). The hallucinations generally consist of persecutory voices that talk about the patient in the third person and comment on the patient's behavior. Blocking, neologisms, perseveration, and disturbed syntax are quite common. Simultaneously, affect is usually warm and friendly or irritable and depressed rather than prototypically schizophrenic.

In addition, other researchers (e.g., Flor-Henry, 1969) have found that untreated, left lateralized CPS manifests itself in a schizophrenia-like psychosis under stress and over time and that untreated, right lateralized or bilateral CPS manifests itself as a psychotic depressive or bipolar disorder under stress or over time. Kristensen and Sindrup (1978) found results like those of Flor-Henry and also found that CPS patients exhibiting psychosis had a lower frequency of seizures than those not exhibiting psychosis; they found that the psychosis developed late (median of 18 years for onset of psychosis after CPS). Others (Toone, 1982; Trimble, 1978; also see Bibliography) have found left lateralization associated with a schizophrenia-like psychosis and bilateral CPS with bipolar-like psychosis.

Some unknown, but we suspect large, number of people diagnosed as schizophrenic may be cases of CPS. Because CPS can be caused by injury during delivery or by anoxia at birth and prolonged, high fevers as an infant, many people who grew up poor and without adequate medical care and appear to be schizophrenic (as adults 20-40 years later) are likely to have CPS (or temporal lobe tumors).

Finally, as noted previously, treating these symptoms with antipsychotics and antidepressants increases and exacerbates the symptoms such that the ostensible schizophrenic appears to be deteriorating. This is because these patients are not schizophrenics; they are epileptics, and the proper treatment for their symptoms is an anticonvulsant. Antipsychotics and antidepressants have been demonstrated to evoke slow electrical activity and therefore can elicit and encourage seizures (Toone & Fenton, 1977; Trimble, 1978, see References).

Summary

Complex partial seizure disorder has many faces and can be misdiagnosed as depression, bipolar disorder, schizophrenia, somatization, hysteria, fugue, multiple personality disorder, anxiety disorder, hypochondria, sexual disorders, or personality disorders. Thus, it is extremely important that therapists screen all patients (especially women who seem to be depressed, anxious, hysterical, and hypochondriacal or to have a borderline personality disorder) for this disorder. In appendix B, we describe simple questions that will assist therapists in ruling out CPS.

References

Bear, D. (1979a). Temporal lobe epilepsy: A syndrome of sensory-limbic hyperconnection. *Cortex, 15,* 357-384.

Bear, D. (1979b). The temporal lobes: An approach to the study of organic behavioral changes. In M. Gazzaniga (Ed.), *Handbook of behavioral neurobiology, and neuropsychology.* New York: Plenum.

Bear, D., & Fedio, P. (1977). Quantitative analysis of interictal behavior in temporal lobe epilepsy. *Archives of Neurology, 34,* 454-467.

Benson, D. F., & Blumer D. (Eds.). (1975). *Psychiatric aspects of neurologic disease.* New York: Grune & Stratton.

Berman, A. (1972). Neurological dysfunction in juvenile delinquency: Implications for early intervention. *Child Care Quarterly, 1*(4), 164-271.

Berman, A., & Siegal, A. (1976). A neuropsychological approach to the etiology, prevention, and treatment of juvenile delinquency. In A. Davids (Ed), *Child personality and psychopathology: Current topics* (Vol 3). New York: John Wiley.

Blumer, D. (1971). Neuropsychiatric aspects of psychomotor and other forms of epilepsy. In S. Livingston (Ed.), *Comprehensive management of epilepsy in infancy, childhood, and adolescence.* Springfield, IL: Charles C Thomas.

Blumer, D. (1975). Temporal lobe epilepsy and its psychiatric significance. In D. F. Benson & D. Blumer (Eds.), *Psychiatric aspects of neurologic disease.* New York: Grune & Stratton.

Blumer, D. (1976). Epilepsy and violence. In D. J. Madder & J. Lion (Eds.), *Rage, hate, assault and other forms of violence.* New York: Spectrum.

Blumer, D. (1977, June). Treatment of patients with seizure disorder referred because of psychiatric complications. *McLean Hospital Journal,* pp. 53-73.

Flor-Henry, P. (1969). Psychosis and temporal lobe epilepsy: A controlled investigation. *Epilepsia, 10,* 363-395.

Hecaen, H., & Albert, M. L. (1978a). Auditory illusions and hallucinations. In H. Hecaen & M. L. Albert (Eds.), *Human neuropsychology* (pp. 257-276). New York: John Wiley.

Hecaen, H., & Albert, M. L. (1978b). Visual illusions and hallucinations. In H. Hecaen & M. L. Albert (Eds.), *Human neuropsychology* (pp. 144-165). New York: John Wiley.

Kristensen, O., & Sindrup, E. H. (1978). Psychomotor epilepsy and psychosis. *Acta Neurologica Scandinavica, 57,* 361-370.

Ounsted, C., & Lindsay, J. (1982). The long-term outcome of temporal lobe epilepsy in childhood. In E. H. Reynolds & M. R. Trimble (Eds.), *Psychiatry and epilepsy* (pp. 185-215). London: Churchill Livingstone.

Slater, E., & Beard, A. W. (1963). The schizophrenia-like psychosis of epilepsy. *British Journal of Psychiatry, 109,* 95-150.

Taylor, J. (1931). *Selected writings of Hughlings Jackson* (Vols. 1 & 2). London: Hodder & Stoughton.

Toone, B. (1982). Psychoses of epilepsy. In E. H. Reynolds & M. R. Trimble (Eds.), *Psychiatry and epilepsy.* London: Churchill Livingstone.

Toone, B. K., & Fenton, G. W. (1977). Epileptic seizures induced by psychotropic drugs. *Psychological Medicine, 7,* 265-270.

Trimble, M. R. (1978). Non-MAOI antidepressants and epilepsy. A review. *Epilepsia, 19,* 241-250.

Weiner, J. H. et al. (1966). An EEG study of delinquents and non-delinquents. *Archives of General Psychiatry, 15,* 144-150.

PART III

Other Disorders

Multiple Sclerosis and Mitral Valve Prolapse

Multiple Sclerosis

The various parts of the brain communicate with each other by sending electrical signals back and forth, and the brain communicates with the body (for example, with the muscles) in the same manner. Many of the nerve tracts or pathways in the brain and spinal cord are covered with a protective covering called *myelin*. The myelin sheath is much like the insulation that covers the electrical wires in one's home. This myelin sheath feeds nutrients to the nerves within it and controls the passage of electrical impulses along the nerves. When the myelin sheath becomes swollen or deteriorates, the condition is called multiple sclerosis (MS). This deterioration and loss of myelin through-out the brain and nervous system are much like randomly and haphazardly stripping off sections of the insulation of the wiring in one's home: Electrical impulses (messages from brain to body), like electricity in one's home, then flow in wild and random ways, increasing, decreasing, and short-circuiting and resulting in a host of psychiatric and physical symptoms. Typical neurons, with an inset highlighting the myelin sheath, are shown in Figure 8.1

The cause of this neurological disease remains unknown. Many regard it as an *autoimmune disorder*. That classification, however, tells us only the *how,* the process of the disease, and sheds no light on the *why,* the cause of the disease. We do know, however, that MS tends to appear most often in cold climates and almost never in warm or tropical ones. Thus, it is far more prevalent in the higher latitudes of the northern and southern hemispheres, with *no cases* of MS found between the latitudes of 40 degrees north and 40

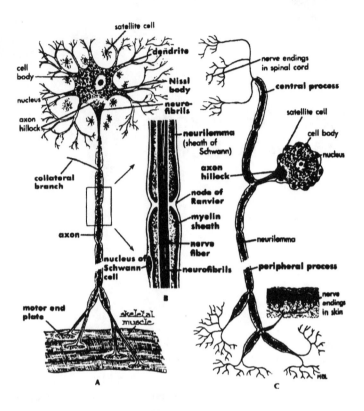

Figure 8.1. Neurons, With Panel Showing Myelin Sheath

SOURCE: From *Functional Human Anatomy* (2nd ed.), by J. E. Crouch, 1972, p. 480. Philadelphia: Lea & Febiger. Reprinted with permission.

degrees south. Instead, it appears among those born above the 40th parallel, which runs through downtown Boulder, Colorado. Therefore, the disease tends to be found among those who live in the northern United States and in northern countries (as well as the northern sections of those countries) throughout the world. If those born above the 40th parallel move below it early in their childhoods, their rate of MS decreases to nearly that of those born below the 40th parallel. The reasons for this epidemiological distribution remain unknown.

MS is also significantly more likely to occur among people of Western European descent than of Eastern or Southern European descent. Thus, MS is more common among Germans, Scandinavians, and Anglo-Saxons than among Italians, Jews, and the Spanish. It is, in this sense, a "White" disease. It almost never occurs in Asians, Asian Americans, or African Americans and does not exist among Africans (because the entire continent of Africa falls between the latitudes of 40 degrees north and 40 degrees south). Finally, MS is significantly more common among women than among men and appears in women between the ages of 20 and 40 years (it is a disease of young adult women). It does not appear in children or in people over 60. Thus, MS is a young, northern, White woman's disease, for reasons that remain unknown. It is clearly not hereditary, however.

Because myelin is widespread throughout the body, the symptoms of MS can take a variety of forms. Neurologically, there is no "classic" form of the disease, except that the diversity of symptoms always waxes and wanes, with symptom-saturated and symptom-free weeks or months. Each exacerbation or symptom-saturated episode is worse than the one before it, so the disease is progressive in this sense. Despite the differences in the symptoms exhibited, however, it is typical for MS to affect the optic nerves, cerebellum, and portions of the spinal cord first. Thus, the patient will complain of tingling or numbness in one spot or limb or side of the body; of temporary weakness, clumsiness, and ataxia (especially after a hot bath or exercise); and of occasional blurred vision. Generally, however, these neurological signs are not apparent until *late in the disease,* and typically, the neurological etiology is not evident until late in the disease.

Instead, in its early states (the first 5 or 10 years of the disease) the symptoms of MS are purely psychological and appear hysterical in the classic sense of the term. These psychiatric symptoms not only add to the problem of accurate diagnosis of MS but also require therapy.

At the beginning of the disease, there tends to be euphoria, a general happiness and high spirits accompanied by exaggerated affect. This intense, exaggerated emotional display and generalized euphoria, particularly if associated with the hypersexuality often seen in MS, looks histrionic, hypomanic, cyclothymic, or bipolar and is typically misdiagnosed as one of these psychiatric disorders. This euphoria, apparent histrionics, and emotional lability are not related to some underlying, premorbid personality disorder. Instead, the degree of euphoria and histrionics is directly predicted by the extent of demyelination (loss of myelin).

Euphoria, ostensible hypomania, and histrionics are not the only affective face of MS. Rather, many patients instead exhibit severe depression with suicidal ideation. As a rule, MS patients score higher than normal and higher than neurological controls on the Minnesota Multiphasic Personality Inventory (MMPI) Scale 2 as well as on the Beck Depression Inventory. Because they score significantly higher on measures of depression than matched, neurological controls (who have muscular dystrophy or amyotrophic lateral sclerosis), it is clear that the depressive symptoms seen in MS are not simply a reaction to having a degenerative, neurological disease nor a reaction to hearing such a diagnosis. In studies in which patients with MS and complex partial seizure (CPS) disorder are compared with patients with other neurological disorders, MS patients and CPS patients exhibit the greatest number of depressive symptoms and significantly more of these than the neurological control groups. For the CPS patients, as we saw in the last chapter, these symptoms are the signs of seizures in the temporal lobes. For MS patients, these depressive symptoms are the result of progressive, rapid, demyelination of the temporal lobes and thalamus.

Thus, what appears to be a prototypical neurotic or psychotic depression is one of the most common faces of MS. *Suicide risk in MS patients is about 14 times higher than that of the general population.* Because MS is a young, White woman's disease and depression and histrionic personality disorder are most common in that population, numerous ostensibly depressed or histrionic White women may represent misdiagnosed cases of MS.

Other, less common faces of MS include a rapid-cycling, ostensible bipolar disorder with classic hypomanic and depressive episodes; an unclassifiable psychosis with hypersexuality and visual hallucinations; and a sudden dementia with rapid deterioration of all cognitive functions. Each of these faces of MS represents the rapid demyelination of the temporal lobes and other brain areas, such as the frontal lobes.

On neuropsychological tests, MS patients exhibit deficits in perceptual-motor skills, abstraction, and memory. On the Wechsler Adult Intelligence Scale (WAIS) this appears early as low scores on Object Assembly, Digit Symbol, Digit Span, and Similarities subscales. Usually, overlearned language skills (Vocabulary, Information, and Comprehension subscales) are preserved. Although the MS patient's problems with perceptual-motor tasks might be an artifact of weakness and ataxia (with subsequent difficulty on WAIS Performance subtests), the difficulties in abstraction and memory cannot similarly be dismissed; these difficulties represent demyelination of various portions of the brain, the temporal lobes in particular. Such cognitive impairment is best predicted by the length of the disease.

Physical symptoms help differentiate MS from psychiatric disturbances. These include ataxia, weakness, numbness and tingling sensations, and urinary incontinence. However, if the patient's presentation is euphoria-emotional-lability-hypersexuality such that she is misdiagnosed as hysterical, these physical symptoms of MS can be similarly misattributed to histrionics and somatization.

Emotional stress, dehydration, changes in calcium levels, and heat can elicit and exacerbate the symptoms of MS. Heat, in particular, increases the symptoms of MS. The reason is that nerves already damaged by the loss of their myelin are very sensitive to even the slightest increases in temperature, because these increases make it nearly impossible for communication within the body and between the body and brain to occur. Thus, one safe and reliable method of screening patients for MS is known as the "hot bath test." The patient is asked to go home and take a nice, hot bath and to observe what happens to her immediately following this bath. In patients who have yet to exhibit any neurological symptoms, extreme weakness and severe, uncontrollable ataxia will result from the hot bath. Such ataxia is prototypical of MS and does not appear in histrionic, manic-depressive, psychotic, or depressed patients and so is a good, differential diagnostic sign.

One of the treatments for MS involves the use of adrenocorticotropic hormone (ACTH). Although ACTH often decreases the neurological symptoms of MS, in many patients, it also increases the euphoria and emotional lability, and in approximately 10% of patients, it precipitates a psychosis.

Until recently, there was no way to definitively confirm the diagnosis of MS other than to find evidence of demyelinization at autopsy. However, the advent of magnetic resonance imaging (MRI) has changed that. During an MRI evaluation, the person is placed inside a large circular magnet that causes the hydrogen atoms found in the body to move. When the magnet is turned off, the hydrogen atoms return to their original positions. This causes an electromagnetic signal that can be read by a computer and then translated into a picture of the internal structures. Patients with MS show a characteristic pattern of demyelinization that appears as white patches on the MRI. Thus, if the hot bath test of a woman who seems histrionic, depressed, or both is positive and MS is therefore suspected, the woman should be referred to a neurologist for an MRI evaluation.

A Case Example: Carol

Carol was a 26-year-old White woman referred for management and treatment of depression from the neurology service to one of the authors (in the behavioral medicine clinic). She gave the following history. At about age 17, she ran away from home because she felt her parents were too restrictive. For the next 5 years or so, she led a rather wild life, becoming involved with drugs, engaging in random sexual encounters, and so forth. Some time around age 22 or 23, she'd had enough of this lifestyle and decided to seek assistance. She saw many therapists during this time, all of whom focused on her rebelliousness, histrionics, and her "poor impulse control." She joined a church, finished high school, and started classes at a junior college. At that time, she began to experience episodes of muscular weakness and anesthesia. These symptoms were attributed by her various therapists to the guilt that she supposedly felt about her prior lifestyle and about her poor relationship with her parents.

Despite the intervention of numerous psychotherapists, her symptoms progressed rapidly, such that within 1 year after her lifestyle change she was confined to a wheelchair. At that time, the diagnosis of MS was made. By the time she was seen by one of the authors 2 years later, the disease had progressed to the point where she was unable to move anything below her neck. She was extremely depressed at that time, and she resented the involvement of the many therapists, all of whom had failed to suggest she obtain a neurological consultation. She felt punished for her decision to change her lifestyle and repeatedly asked why this had to happen to her now, when she had attempted to make her life better. She was suicidal and often complained that her inability to move her arms even took the option of suicide away from her. Her periods of remission were short-lived and rarely amounted to anything more than a slight increase in arm or leg mobility. She now required skilled nursing care and resided permanently at a nursing home. Although the new friends she had made from church since her change in lifestyle continued to provide her with some social support, she never made amends with her family. She was repeatedly admitted to the hospital every 2 or 3 months for urinary tract infections and other problems that were the result of her MS and her paralysis; during each of these admissions, she was seen for brief problem-oriented psychotherapy.

Thus, the correct neurological diagnosis was not made for many years. Had it been made when she was young and involved in her "wild" lifestyle, she might have had the opportunity to change that lifestyle (itself a symptom of MS) and live a fuller life as well as reconcile with her family prior to her deterioration. In addition, even after the correct physical diagnosis had been made, there was still the need for psychological intervention. This is true for many, if not most, MS patients, who need to learn to cope with the specific limitations of their disease. Likewise, psychological intervention for close friends and family is also often warranted because the disease has a tremendous impact on significant others.

Interim Summary

MS is a disease of White women aged 20 to 40 that can readily be misdiagnosed as neurotic or psychotic depression, bipolar disorder, histrionic personality disorder, conversion disorder, or atypical psychosis, with depression (Axis I) and hysterical personality (Axis II) being the most common misdiagnoses. The "hot bath test" as well as a WAIS (on which a low score on the Similarities subscale appears), along with information about where the patient was born, can help differentiate this neurological disorder from psychopathology. In addition, MRI testing can confirm the suspected diagnosis of MS.

Mitral Valve Prolapse

A variety of anxiety-related and panic symptoms have been associated with problems in the cardiovascular system, which includes the heart and all of the veins and arteries that transport blood throughout the body. These cardiovascular disorders can be misdiagnosed as anxiety disorders, with mitral valve prolapse foremost among those. Here, we briefly describe the structure and functions of the heart and the mitral valve and how and why mitral valve prolapse can be misdiagnosed as a panic disorder.

The heart is a pump that consists of four chambers. Figure 8.2 shows the inside of the heart, with the four chambers noted as RA = right atrium, RV = right ventricle, LA = left atrium, and LV = left ventricle. Deoxygenated blood (that is, blood that has already traveled through the body and delivered oxygen and other necessary nutrients to the various cells) is carried back to the heart through a system of veins ending in the venae cavae. This blood flows directly into the RA. Most of the blood that enters the RA then flows passively into the RV through the tricuspid valve. When the RV is full, the tricuspid valve closes, the RV contracts, and blood is propelled into the pulmonary artery. This artery carries the blood to the lungs, where the blood again receives the necessary oxygen to carry back to the body. This oxygenated blood then travels through the pulmonary veins into the LA of the heart. From the LA, the blood passes through the mitral valve to the LV. When the LV is full, the mitral valve closes, the LV contracts, and the oxygenated blood is then propelled to the rest of the body through the aorta. Oxygenated blood travels through a system of increasingly smaller and smaller arteries and arterioles to the capillaries, where the oxygen and other nutrients actually enter the cells and carbon dioxide and waste metabolites leave. The now deoxygenated blood then travels through a series of increasingly larger venules and veins until it reaches the venae cavae, which returns it to the RA of the heart.

The period when the heart muscles are relaxed and blood entering the atria flows passively into the ventricles through the open tricuspid and mitral valves is called *diastole*. When the pressure in the ventricles becomes greater than the pressure in the atria, these two valves close, which generates the first heart sound. The period when the ventricles contract and blood is propelled into either the pulmonary arteries or the aorta is called *systole*. Following this contraction, the valves to both the pulmonary artery and the aorta close,

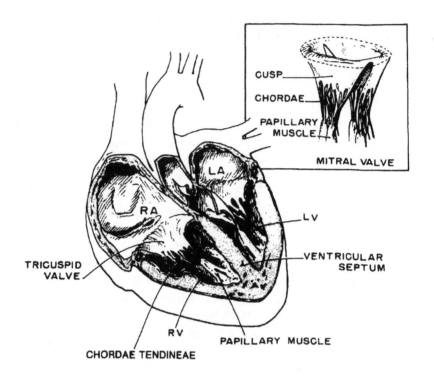

Figure 8.2. Structures of the Heart

SOURCE: From *Pathophysiology: Clinical concepts of disease processes* (4th ed.), by S. A. Price and L. M. Wilson, 1992, p. 374, St. Louis, MO: Mosby Year Book, Inc.

causing the second heart sound. This is then again followed by the diastole period. One might be familiar with these terms because they are associated with blood pressure: The diastolic blood pressure is the pressure produced by the blood in your system when your heart is at rest and the ventricles are passively filling; the systolic blood pressure is the pressure when your heart is contracting and sending blood throughout your body. This is why systolic pressure is greater than diastolic pressure.

In mitral valve prolapse (MVP), for reasons that are unknown, the mitral valve bows back into the LA during systole (prolapse). For reasons that also are unknown, this condition is often experienced by the person with MVP as the heart suddenly racing (or frequently racing) and so is misinterpreted by the individual experiencing it as anxiety or as a sudden panic attack. Consequently, about 8% of MVP patients report panic attacks and about 20% of people with panic disorders have been found to have MVP. In other studies, 30% of patients with generalized anxiety disorder and 44% of patients with bipolar affective disorder were discovered to have MVP. Although these data at first suggest a strong relationship between MVP and anxiety disorders and therefore imply that MVP may be frequently misdiagnosed as anxiety disorder, other data are not consistent with these findings.

For example, the estimated prevalence of MVP has ranged from 4% to 21%, depending on the population studied and on the manner in which MVP was diagnosed. When diagnosed using a stethoscope (a procedure called *auscultation*) rates of MVP are high, and this was often the diagnostic procedure in early studies. When diagnosed through the new procedure of echocardiography (during which sound is used to image the various internal structures of the heart, allowing visualization and measurement of the mitral valve), rates of MVP are lower. In addition, many early studies that found a strong relationship between anxiety disorders and MVP were not done "blind"; the physicians diagnosing the MVP knew that the patient had panic attacks, and the physicians diagnosing the panic attacks knew that the patient had MVP, and this knowledge could have biased the findings. Likewise, the criteria for diagnosing MVP were highly variable (particularly in early studies), and the use of the published guidelines remains subjective and varies from study to study. The best studies suggest that the overall prevalence of MVP is 3% to 4% but that there are striking age and gender effects: For men, the prevalence of MVP is 2% to 4% at all ages; for women, *the rate of MVP was 17% for those between the ages of 20 and 29,* but less than 2% for those over age 70. The reason for these gender and age differences in this cardiac disorder are unknown. Panic attacks, similarly, occur relatively often and occur primarily among young women.

What do these conflicting results mean for the practicing clinician? These data certainly suggest that some (young) women who present generalized anxiety or panic attacks may have MVP and imply that MVP might be responsible for their symptoms. Thus, every patient who presents with panic or generalized anxiety disorder should be asked about prior cardiac history. Specifically, she should be asked if she has ever been told that she had a benign heart murmur or that there were extra heart sounds. Most cases of MVP are not thought to be serious or life threatening, and as a result, many physicians merely note the problem without treating it. If your patient reports that she has been told that she has a murmur, a reevaluation, usually including an echocardiogram, is warranted. Although one can never actually prove that the MVP is causing the panic attacks and anxiety, many patients are relieved to hear that their "psychiatric" problem may have a physical substrate; being able to attribute their "anxiety" to a cardiac disorder helps them understand and adjust to their symptoms. Therapists can assist patients in reattributing the anxiety to the cardiac problem, and this can lead to improvements in mood. Nonetheless, psychotherapeutic treatment of the anxiety is still required and should be conducted in the standard manner.

A Case Example: Miriam

Miriam was a 24-year-old married Orthodox Jewish woman who presented with a chief complaint of severe agoraphobia with panic. The problem began approximately a year before being seen. Initially, the problem consisted of vague feelings of anxiety and panic that occurred whenever Miriam went out of the house. Over a 6-month period, these had increased in both frequency and intensity such that her husband, Lenny, increasingly was asked to be more responsible for the day-to-day tasks that Miriam had previously handled, such as running errands, shopping, taking their daughter to the doctor, and so forth. Miriam had been to see her internist a number of times about the problem. He had prescribed 5 mg of Valium to be taken once or twice a day. However, as the symptoms worsened, Miriam began taking more and more Valium. At the time of her initial evaluation, she was taking four to five Valiums per day, despite the fact that she reported that they did not really help with the anxiety. She also began to feel depressed because she felt she was not living up to her role as wife and mother. She was not actively suicidal, but she had begun to have some thoughts of ending her life. Although her internist had suggested that she seek counseling, both she and her husband were against the idea, in part because they felt their religious beliefs were not especially supportive of psychological treatment. They eventually sought treatment, however, after a particularly bad experience. Miriam had been at the grocery store to do the week's shopping. While there, she experienced such severe panic that she had to run from the store, leaving all of her groceries in the cart in the middle of the aisle and barely remembering to take her 3-year-old child with her (she had to go back and get the child). After this, she refused to do any task that involved leaving the house. Because her husband felt overwhelmed by the housekeeping responsibilities in addition to his job, he discussed Miriam's condition with his rabbi. After much debate and discussion, the rabbi concluded that Miriam's situation was indeed desperate, and he reluctantly gave his blessing to their seeking treatment.

Miriam had an interesting psychosocial history. She was one of three daughters. She reported that she was the one most often picked on by her parents. She described a very intrusive relationship in which her parents often told her what to do and how to do it. At about age 18 she met Lenny. Although she was not herself raised in an Orthodox Jewish household, she began to study Orthodox Judaism to prepare herself to marry Lenny, who was himself very Orthodox. Thus, she spent significant time learning how to keep a kosher kitchen, learning the rituals surrounding the various holidays and celebrations in the Jewish calendar, learning about appropriate ways Orthodox wives should behave and dress, and so forth. Soon, she was sufficiently culturally prepared that she was able to marry Lenny. Although she reported that the other Orthodox women were nice to her, she somehow felt as if she did not really belong. In addition, although she went along with the Orthodox lifestyle, covering her head whenever she went out of her house and keeping all of the rules and regulations to the best of her ability, to herself she often questioned the value of such activities. She privately wondered if she had made a mistake marrying Lenny and joining the Orthodox community so quickly. Within the first few years of marriage she got pregnant. Her 3-year-old daughter further contributed to her rarely acknowledged feelings of being trapped in something she was no longer sure was right for her.

Miriam and Lenny both came to the initial evaluation session. As would be expected, questions directed toward Miriam were usually answered by Lenny. Miriam merely sat and sighed repeatedly. Lenny described in detail the hardships and burdens being placed on him by his wife's symptoms. Although acknowledging that during the periods of panic his wife was clearly upset, Lenny's underlying message seemed to be that Miriam was just not trying hard enough. He seemed to have very little empathy or understanding of the degree to which Miriam herself experienced these episodes as distressing. It quickly became clear that Miriam would not speak for herself as long as Lenny remained in the room, so the therapist asked to speak with Miriam alone.

Once alone, she described the following symptoms. Whenever she needed to leave the house, she experienced increased anxiety in anticipation of going out. Once she left, however, within 1 hour, these feelings of anxiety escalated and manifested themselves in a physical way. She reported increased heart rate, faster breathing, and feeling as if she were going to have a heart attack. Once these symptoms began, she felt they would not go away until she was able to return to her house. Thus, she would stop whatever she was doing and return home immediately. As a result, she never forced herself to tolerate these uncomfortable feelings to see if they would eventually go away on their own. She took the Valium both prophylactically, to prevent the feelings from starting, and symptomatically, to stop the feelings once they began. At the time of her evaluation, the feelings of panic were no longer limited to times when she left the house. Rather, the increases in anxiety were occurring about four or five times a day.

During this evaluation, Miriam was asked a number of routine questions about her prior medical history. According to her, during her first gynecological examination, she was told by the gynecologist that she had an extra heart sound, a "benign murmur" that did not require any additional evaluation or treatment. The thought of this murmur would often come to her during the panic attacks, further fueling her fear that she was having a heart attack.

The initial treatment began along two lines simultaneously. Miriam would be seen individually, without Lenny, until the panic symptoms were under better control. As a first step to achieving this, Miriam was asked to keep detailed records of her anxiety. These records included what was happening when she felt the anxiety, a rating (on a 1 to 10 scale) of the severity of the anxiety, and what she did (or did not do) because of the anxiety. In addition, she was asked to record each time she took a Valium or did anything else that she thought would decrease her anxiety. Concurrently, she was referred for an echocardiogram to evaluate the possibility that she had mitral valve prolapse.

Within 2 weeks, the results of the echocardiogram had demonstrated that Miriam indeed had mitral valve prolapse. The mitral valve prolapse was not, however, sufficiently severe as to require either medication or any other medical intervention. The potential implications of this diagnosis with respect to the panic attacks she was experiencing were explained to her. She was told that, although this was not a life-threatening condition, she did have a more labile autonomic nervous system than other people. Because her nervous system was more labile (more reactive), she was more likely to experience change in heart rate, change in breathing, and increased perspiration. These changes could occur randomly, unpredictably, frequently, and apparently without cause. That meant that the feelings of panic might be occurring because of this nervous system lability and as a result she was misattributing this lability as anxiety. It was explained to her that the uncomfortable feelings would eventually pass, regardless of what she herself did about them.

Simultaneously, from the records she was keeping it was clear that the experience of anxiety was often being reinforced: She would experience an increase in the anxiety whenever she was confronted with tasks that she preferred to avoid (e.g., seeing Lenny's parents), and frequently, she was able to avoid these things because of the anxiety (this reinforced the anxiety). The onset and termination of the anxiety were random cardiac events, however; the anxiety did not begin *because* of the unpleasant task and did not end *because* she avoided the task (it ended because it had run its course). But Miriam *thought* that the anxiety was associated with certain tasks and so avoided or escaped from those. Fear of specific places and tasks therefore was learned in a manner matching the acquisition of agoraphobia in people who have no cardiac disorder—despite the fact that her anxiety actually was unrelated to the places and tasks in question. Thus, again, a patient's explanation for her physical symptoms (that these were caused by certain situations rather than by her heart) played a role in her psychiatric problems. In this case, the misattribution of anxiety to situations led to the acquisition of agoraphobia. The standard treatment for agoraphobia, based on exposure and response prevention, thus was appropriate.

A list of the usual situations Miriam might find herself in was prepared. This included events such as going to her daughter's preschool, taking her daughter to the doctor, attending synagogue, visiting friends, visiting various relatives, going out to eat, shopping in a wide range of different kinds of stores, and so forth. Using the records Miriam had been keeping as well as her own observations of these situations, a hierarchy was developed. All of the situations were ranked from least panic producing to most panic producing. The rationale behind the treatment was explained to Miriam. She was informed that part of the reason the panic had increased in frequency was that when the panic began, she escaped from the situation. It was noted that in reality the feelings she called anxiety would go away one way or another: That is, she could either leave the situation or wait and eventually the feelings of panic would dissipate on their own. Leaving the situation served only to reinforce the panic, so it was necessary to train herself to remain in various situations despite how she was feeling. She was instructed to remind herself of the mitral valve prolapse whenever she began to experience panic. In other words, she was told to say to herself, "This is not really anxiety. This is only my mitral valve prolapse and my labile nervous system that is making me feel this way. I am not having a heart attack nor am I dying. These feelings are not related to where I am right now or to what I am doing right now. If I wait long enough, eventually I will begin to feel better on my own." These phrases were written on a sheet of paper that Miriam carried with her to be read when necessary and helped her label her symptoms correctly and make the right attributions for them.

Beginning with the situations at the low end of the hierarchy (least likely to produce anxiety and panic), Miriam was then assigned to put herself in those situations. She was instructed to place herself in no fewer than two of the situations per day. Once she entered each situation, she was instructed that she could not leave until she either finished what she came to do or the anxiety had gone away on its own. Should panic begin, she was instructed to take out the piece of paper describing the role of her mitral valve prolapse and read it until the episode passed. In addition, she was to tell herself that the panic and anxiety would soon be over. The importance of not escaping from the situation was stressed repeatedly, and the potential negative impact of escape as she made progress was also explained.

Over the next 8 to 10 weeks, Miriam exposed herself to the situations on her list in a systematic, hierarchical, and organized way. As she did so, the frequency and intensity of her panic decreased. Because the treatment for the panic was so straightforward, very little therapy time was necessary to deal with symptoms of anxiety other than to review her progress from week to week and help her decide how to take the next step in the situation hierarchy. This left time to discuss her relationship with her husband, her feelings about being Orthodox, her relationship with her parents, and so forth. During the course of treatment, she decided to remove her head covering and discuss some of her concerns with Lenny. A number of sessions were devoted to working with both partners together to improve the relationship and make Miriam a more equal partner. By the end of treatment, Miriam was able to go anywhere and stay as long as necessary without being overcome by panic. In addition, she and Lenny had made significant progress in improving the nature and quality of their relationship. Miriam felt more in control, was less depressed, and was more confident in her abilities as a wife and mother. She was considering going back to school and obtaining training that would enable her to work once her child was older.

The diagnosis of mitral valve prolapse greatly facilitated Miriam's treatment by providing an acceptable attribution for the uncomfortable and distressing symptoms she was experiencing. This attribution was then used in the exposure and response prevention treatment to enable her to remain in situations in which she felt panic. The relative ease with which the panic attacks were treated allowed therapy time to be devoted to important marital and cultural issues and ensured that all aspects of Miriam's life were improved as a result of therapy.

Systemic Lupus Erythematosus (SLE) and Other Disorders

Systemic Lupus Erythematosus

The immunological system of the human body specializes in differentiating self from not-self. When something appears in the body that is not-self, such as a virus, bacterium, or transplanted organ, the immunological system recognizes the alien as such and sets out to destroy it. This system works very well and is our first line of defense against disease, although its tendency to lead to the rejection of transplanted organs remains problematic. Precisely how the immunologic system recognizes and differentiates self from not-self is not clear. Sometimes, for reasons that also are not understood, the immunological system makes a big mistake in that differentiation. In these cases, the immunological system mistakenly identifies the body and its parts as not-self and then attacks and destroys them. When this happens, the disorder in question is called an autoimmune disorder (where *auto* = *self*). Systemic lupus erythematosus (SLE or simply *lupus*) is an autoimmune disorder in which the immunologic system attacks the body and the brain (the cerebral cortex and basil ganglia in particular). Graves' disease (Chapter 2) and multiple sclerosis (Chapter 7) are now also regarded as autoimmune disorders, and some data strongly suggest that 50% of cases of Addison's disease (Chapter 2) are autoimmune disorders.

Lupus (which means *wolf* in Latin) was so named because of the color of its characteristic rash by Ferdinand von Hebra in 1845. Throughout the late 1800s, it was incessantly misdiagnosed as a dermatological (skin) disease and then as a form of tuberculosis, until the famed dermatologist Moritz Kaposi, chair of the Department of Dermatology at the Vienna University Hospital, recognized its systemic nature. Today, it is likely to be misdiagnosed not as a dermatological disorder but as psychopathology.

Lupus is a common disease that strikes more than 1 in every 2,000 people; some estimate that *1 million people per year* develop this disease with only half of these diagnosed correctly. *Of its victims, 85% to 90% are women, who outnumber men with the disorder at the rate of 10 to 1.* The women most likely to have lupus are between the ages of 20 and 50 years, with African American and Native American women more likely to have this disease than women of other ethnic groups, at a ratio of approximately 3 to 1. Thus, just as multiple sclerosis (MS) is a White woman's disease for the most part, lupus is, for the most part, an African American and a Native American woman's disease.

Because the brain is being attacked and destroyed by the immunological system, lupus presents in a host of psychiatric symptoms that are insidious in onset and likely to be misdiagnosed as psychopathology. In many cases, these symptoms represent simple and complex focal seizures caused by the immunological system's attacks on the brain. Classic, prototypical depressive symptoms are the most common face of lupus, appearing in 66% of patients. Fatigue, weight loss, and severe anorexia nervosa typically appear with the depressive symptoms and only increase the probability of psychiatric misdiagnosis. Lupus is associated with arthritis in 45% to 90% of the patients and with migraine headaches in nearly 100% of patients, but these physical symptoms can be misinterpreted as the somatization seen in depression or are ignored as irrelevant to the symptom picture. Thus, lupus is most likely to be misdiagnosed as depression, anorexia nervosa, or both and may account for some large but unknown percentage of cases of these disorders among African American and Native American women. Questioning ostensibly depressed or anorectic women about migraines and arthritis can be useful in ruling out this physical disorder.

Other faces of lupus include the following:

- A psychotic thought disorder with hallucinations and delusions that is difficult to distinguish from schizophrenia
- Nonspecific, organic brain syndromes with deterioration of cognitive functioning, strokes, and identifiable focal seizures
- An episodic dyscontrol syndrome characterized by sudden rage and violence

The physical symptoms of lupus are equally slow and insidious in onset and thus may increase rather than decrease psychiatric misdiagnosis. These include episodic joint and muscle pain, cough, fever, migraine headaches, arthritis, and chest or heart pain, along with nausea, and morning stiffness. If the patient smokes, as many African American women do, the coughing, chest pain, and heart pain can be dismissed as the consequence of smoking. Hypertension, anemia, and hepatitis are also common and can readily be dismissed as typical of African American and Native American women (hypertension, anemia) or dismissed as unrelated to the ostensible psychiatric symptoms (hepatitis). Other patients also exhibit photosensitivity (sensitivity to sunlight) and loss of scalp hair. Still others develop ulcerative sores on the nose, mouth, and genitals that can readily be misdiagnosed as a venereal disease. This is because (a) the autoantibodies (chemicals produced to attack the body once it has been mistakenly identified as not-self) lead to false positive syphilis results (i.e., the test indicates that a woman who does not have syphilis does have it) and because (b) racism may predispose physicians to suspect venereal diseases among African American and Native American women.

Like MS, the symptoms of lupus are exacerbated by stress. Theoretically, this is because the immunological system, which becomes very active during stress in all people, becomes active in patients with lupus or MS who are under stress as well. However, because their immunological systems are attacking their myelin (MS) and body and brain (lupus), the increased activity associated with stress may result in an increase in such attacks on the body and so in more severe symptoms. That the symptoms increase when under stress may only further bias therapists toward a mistaken psychological attribution and explanation.

The prototypical physical symptom of lupus is a rash across the nose, but it can be found elsewhere. This can serve as a differential diagnostic sign, provided that it is present, for it occurs somewhere on the body in only 70% of patients. The other physical symptoms mentioned earlier can be differential diagnostic signs if one asks about these and recognizes them as signs and aspects of lupus.

Lupus is a "well controllable disease provided it is recognized early and treated appropriately" (Smolen & Zielinksi, 1987, p. 170) with nonsteroidal, anti-inflammatory drugs (NSAIDS) and other similar drugs (e.g., immuno-suppressants). If it is misdiagnosed and treated as psychopathology, the patient will continue to deteriorate because the disease is progressive and because psychotropic medications either do not help or precipitate additional symptoms. Indeed, there is good evidence that the following drugs not only exacerbate the symptoms of lupus but *can cause* lupus:

- Thorazine
- Antihypertensive drugs (drugs for hypertension)

- Carbamazepine (Tegretol, used to treat seizures, complex partial seizures in particular)
- Antibiotics, such as penicillin and streptomycin
- Succinimides, such as Milontin and Zarontin
- Other anticonvulsants, such as Dilantin (phenytoin)

We cannot estimate how many cases of lupus among African American women have been caused by the use of certain antihypertensive drugs to treat the hypertension that is common in that population, and we cannot estimate how many cases of lupus have been caused by the tendency of ghetto physicians to overprescribe antibiotics to poor African Americans. Likewise, we cannot estimate how many of these iatrogenic cases of lupus among poor African American women are then subsequently misdiagnosed as schizophrenia—a diagnosis this group receives frequently.

Lupus must be considered a possibility in cases of ostensible depression, schizophrenia, organic brain syndrome, conversion disorder, hysteria, somatization, and anorexia nervosa among women—African American and Native American women in particular. Differential diagnostic signs include the presence of the following physical symptoms: arthritis, migraine headaches, chronic cough, chest pain, muscle stiffness, and ulcerative sores. For a personal report of a harrowing struggle to receive an accurate diagnosis of lupus after years of psychotherapy and physical tests, we suggest *Lupus: My Search for a Diagnosis,* by Eileen Radziunas (1989).

Posterolateral Sclerosis

Posterolateral sclerosis is a neurological disorder whose symptoms are severe anxiety and complaints of weakness, numbness, and the sensation that the limbs are heavy. These symptoms can be misdiagnosed as an anxiety disorder. *Stocking and/or glove sensory loss also is common* (loss of feeling in the area that would be covered by a glove or stocking) and can to the misdiagnosis of conversion disorder. As the disease progresses, unambiguously physical symptoms (such as alterations in reflexes) appear, along with memory impairment and psychosis. The disease involves a progressive degeneration of the lateral and posterior columns of the spinal cord and peripheral nerves. Although the gender distribution of this disease is unknown, its anxiety and glove anesthesia are readily mistaken for classic hysteria (conversion disorder); because the latter diagnosis is one that women receive far more often than men, this disorder must be considered a possibility for women exhibiting these symptoms.

Hypoglycemia

As noted earlier, hypoglycemia is abnormally low blood sugar. Normal blood sugar, for which the pancreas is monitoring and adjusting insulin levels for food eaten and energy expended (physical activity), ranges between 80 and 100 mg/100 ml. Severely low blood sugar can result in coma and death. However, there is a middle range, where blood sugar is low but the patient is still functional, and this is known as hypoglycemia. The generally accepted lower limit of the normal range of blood sugar is between 50 and 60 mg/100 ml, although some endocrinologists feel that blood sugar levels above 45 mg/100 ml should not cause symptoms and do not justify the diagnosis of hypoglycemia. Symptoms of hypoglycemia typically include sweating, shakiness, and palpitations, which are often misattributed to anxiety. The diagnosis of hypoglycemia for these symptoms has become quite popular recently, although the lack of agreed-on norms for exactly what constitutes "low" blood sugar remains a problem. Many believe that the diagnosis has been overused and that it is used to explain obscure symptoms because it "gives the patient something to do, i.e., manipulate his or her diet continuously" (Levine, 1974, p. 463). In light of such controversies, it is nonetheless wise to ask patients with symptoms of anxiety about the relationship between the experience of anxiety and when they have eaten most recently. If a fairly consistent pattern is found between mealtime and the symptoms of anxiety, the possibility of hypoglycemia should be considered as an alternative explanation. A single test of blood sugar level to confirm the suspicion of hypoglycemia will not be sufficient, however, and a longer, more intense test is needed. Specifically, patients presenting what appears to be anxiety and suspected of having this disorder (because anxiety is related to when they last ate) should have a 5-hour glucose tolerance test. In this procedure, a fasting patient consumes a specially prepared glucose drink and blood sugar levels are carefully monitored over a 5-hour period of time.

If the patient does have hypoglycemia (confirmed by the test), the symptoms can be easily controlled by having the patient eat four or five small meals a day, with an emphasis on low-carbohydrate foods. In addition, patients may benefit from carrying low-carbohydrate snacks with them to have something to eat if they begin to experience symptoms.

Wilson's Disease (HLD)

Wilson's disease or hepatolenticular degeneration (HLD) is an inherited disorder involving the excessive absorption of copper (from the small intestine), along with decreased excretion of copper by the liver. Copper therefore builds up in the liver and brain, creating psychiatric, neurological, and physical (liver) symptoms. The disease can present purely in psychiatric symptoms, however, without symptoms of basal ganglion degeneration and cirrhosis. The onset is slow and begins between the ages of 11 and 25 years. Early symptoms are episodes of severe anxiety or psychosis, with motoric symptoms (e.g., tremor, gait disturbance, rigidity) appearing later. In children, the disorder is associated with poor grades, speech and language problems, and a behavioral disorder. An amazing diversity of psychiatric symptoms is seen in this disorder, including those that fit the criteria for major depression, schizophrenia, and hysteria in adults and behavioral disorders with school phobia and mental retardation in children. Loss of appetite and weight accompany the psychiatric symptoms seen in adults and increase the tendency to misdiagnose this disease as an anxiety disorder or as a major depressive episode. Hallucinations and delusions also appear and increase the chances of the patient's receiving the misdiagnosis of schizophrenia or psychotic depression. The physical symptoms that assist in differentiating this disease from a psychiatric disturbance do not appear until very late in the disease. These symptoms are signs of liver damage and include cirrhosis and jaundice.

The distribution of this disorder by ethnicity and gender is unknown. Because it commonly presents as depression, anxiety, or hysteria, however, it must be considered a possibility for women exhibiting those symptoms.

Cancer of the Pancreas

The most common face of cancer of the pancreas is severe depression with initial insomnia (difficulty falling asleep), hypersomnia (sleeping too much), and frequent crying spells. Suicidal ideation and severe anxiety are also common. One study of 46 patients with cancer of the pancreas found severe depression in 45 of them; no physical disorder was detected in most of them on preliminary examination.

Unlike the other disorders presented in this book, cancer of the pancreas is seen *more often in men than women,* at a ratio of about 3:1, at age 50 to 70. It can occur in women, however, and so is discussed only briefly. Weight loss, weakness, abdominal pain, severe depression, loss of motivation, and a sense of impending doom are common symptoms. Studies reveal that the depressive symptoms typically were exhibited for 6 months to 4 years prior to the diagnosis of the cancer and were misdiagnosed as functional depression.

Pheochromocytoma

Pheochromocytoma refers to a tumor on the adrenal medulla. Its typical symptoms are attacks of severe anxiety (panic attacks), with sweating, headaches, increased body temperature and appetite, tachycardia, and the other prototypical symptoms of panic disorder. The epidemiological distribution of this disorder is unknown, but its anxiety-related symptoms lead it to warrant consideration.

References

Levine, R. (1974). Hypoglycemia. *JAMA, 230,* 462-463.
Radziunas, E. (1989). *Lupus: My search for a diagnosis* (J. Melvin, Ed.). Claremont, CA: Hunter House.
Smolen, J. S., & Zielinski, C. C. (1987). *Systemic lupus erythematosus.* New York: Springer-Verlag.

PART IV

Clinical Practice
Considerations

10

Interacting With Medical Specialists

A Practical Guide

It is the rare therapist who does not have occasion to deal with medical specialists. Many of us get a significant number of our referrals from physicians. In addition, we make frequent referrals to physicians when or if we suspect some type of underlying physical problem in a patient and when medication may be needed. Indeed, one of the results of this book may be increased interactions with and referrals to physicians, particularly if the reader becomes more sensitive to the possibility that what appears to be psychological may in fact be physical. Rarely do our training programs directly address how best to interact with medical specialists, and most of us develop our interactional style through an arduous process of trial and error. The purpose of this chapter is to describe the types of things that inhibit successful interactions with physicians, methods that can facilitate the interaction, and steps you can take to make your interactions with physicians more helpful to you and your patients.

Inherent Barriers to Communication

One of the first problems in dealing with medical specialists (and these includes physicians, nurses, occupational and physical therapists, and so forth) is the fairly pervasive belief that what psychologists and other therapists do is not really any "big deal" and does not require any specialized training or skills. This misconception derives, in part, from the stereotype of the therapist as a "blank screen" on whom a patient projects her psychopathology without comment or reaction from the therapist. It is further fueled by the erroneous concept that psychotherapy consists primarily of catharsis, which to a layperson (and this includes physicians and other medical specialists) means a process in which the patient "vents" or expresses what she feels to a warm, interested, attentive, and sympathetic listener. The act of venting in and of itself is believed to constitute the entire therapeutic process. In this scenario, all of the work is actually done by the patient; the therapist merely needs to be a good listener. Because practitioners from a variety of other helping professions see themselves as warm, caring, sensitive, and responsive to what a patient says to them, they see themselves as equally able to be good listeners, too. Nursing schools, for example, emphasize that part of being a good nurse is attending to the psychosocial needs of patients, especially listening to what patients say. As a result, there is an often unspoken but nonetheless ever-present underlying belief that *anyone* could do what the mental health professional does because all one has to do is be a good listener. If anyone can "do" therapy, your observations or opinions as a therapist carry little weight and may in fact be viewed as superfluous or unnecessary. Unless you can demonstrate that the treatment you are offering is more than merely "listening," in many medical practitioners' eyes, you are merely replicating what they themselves are providing. This is the first major barrier to communication with medical professionals, demonstrating that the services you offer go beyond merely listening to a patient vent her feelings.

The second major barrier to effective communication is that many medical professionals have little or no respect for or patience with mental health professionals. Some of this lack of respect is the result of the "blank screen" and "good listener" stereotypes discussed above. However, much of it is also the result of negative prior experiences with mental health service providers. For many physicians, their opinion of the value and worth of psychological interventions is shaped during their hospital residency. All too often, a mental health professional is called in to consult on a particularly problematic patient. The patient may be displaying signs of depression, may be noncompliant with the prescribed treatment, may be too demanding of nursing staff time, or may be disruptive to the orderly functioning of the ward. In all of these cases, the patient is a "problem," and the often unspoken but nonetheless very real reason for the referral for mental health services is to have the problem solved. Traditional psychiatric interventions often fail to actively step in and solve the problem. The consultant may merely reconfirm the diagnosis of the problem that led to the referral in the first place. Thus, a patient who appeared depressed to ward staff is indeed diagnosed as "depressed." Or a patient who is disruptive to ward routine is diagnosed as having some type of personality disorder. In either of these cases, the act of making a diagnosis does not solve the problem, and the mental health referral is seen as having been a waste of time. An example might help to clarify this.

Case Example: Linda

The entire nursing staff of a general medical-surgical ward insisted that the resident get someone else to see a particularly troublesome patient after referral to the psychiatric service had not solved the problem. Linda was a 49-year-old African American woman with severe uncontrolled diabetes mellitus. The patient had a long history of failing to comply with her diabetic regimen (i.e., refusing to take her insulin, constantly eating foods that were not allowed on her diabetic diet). She had recently gone blind as a result of the diabetes. She had been admitted to the hospital because her legs had become gangrenous. Gangrene occurs when the blood supply to an area is interrupted for a long period of time and, as a result, the cells in that area die (become necrotic) and are infected with bacteria. Uncontrolled diabetes mellitus can cause disruptions in blood flow (vascular occlusion), with insufficient blood going to a person's extremities; left untreated, gangrene is often the result. Because of the gangrene, Linda's physicians were considering bilateral amputation of her legs. Although she was clearly depressed and needed assistance to become more compliant with her diabetic regimen, the actual reason for the referral was her behavior on the ward: She did not use her call button but, rather, screamed out loudly for nursing assistance at various times (often during the early hours of the morning). Four or five times a day she "fell" out of the bed, even though the bed rails were up and even after being physically restrained. She refused to take her medication (including her insulin) when it was scheduled to be given and then demanded to be given it at later, unpredictable times.

The psychiatrist who saw her a number of times originally diagnosed her as depressed with a borderline personality disorder. He felt that she was grieving for the loss of her physical capabilities and that she was feeling guilty about her current condition because she had not kept to her prescribed diet. Although he prescribed antidepressant medication and met with her a number of times to help her "work through" the guilt and the grieving, after 4 or 5 days she was still screaming for nursing assistance, "falling" out of the bed, and taking her medications whenever she liked. In other words, the referral to psychiatry had not solved the problem, and the problem was the reason for the referral in the first place. Virtually anyone could recognize that she was depressed, and this required no specialized skills. Although the patient might have benefited from therapy to resolve the many issues she had, such therapy would likely take months or years; the hospital staff needed help with this patient immediately.

The treatment approach taken was somewhat unorthodox. After talking with the patient for a long time, it became clear that much of her yelling and falling out of bed was the result of her recent blindness. She was concerned that nursing staff was not checking on her often enough, in part because she could not see if one of them merely poked her head into the room and checked to see if the patient was fine. When she screamed or got out of the bed, she could be certain a nurse was there. Thus, the treatment for these two management problems was done completely by the nursing staff. First, the nurses agreed to check on the patient once each hour at an agreed-on time. Although this was somewhat more frequent than they usually checked on patients, it was felt that the total amount of nursing staff time would eventually be reduced because they would eliminate the random calls for more intensive nursing assistance (e.g., picking her up and putting her back in her bed) at other, less convenient times. During this hourly visit, the nurse was required to converse at least minimally with the patient so that the patient would know the visit had occurred. Because many of the patient's problems occurred during the night, these hourly visits occurred around the clock. If the patient was asleep when the nurse went into the room, the nurse left a tongue depressor on the patient's nightstand as evidence of her visit. Then, if the patient woke during the night and was unsure if she had been checked on, she could merely reach over to her nightstand, pick up the tongue depressors, count them, and know how often a nurse had been there.

To ensure that this was effective, however, nursing staff also had to agree to ignore the patient if she yelled or did anything to call attention to herself in between the regularly scheduled visits. In other words, if the patient "fell" out of the bed, the nurse was instructed to go the patient's room, look in to make sure that she was not injured in any way (but not talking to the patient), and then wait until the next regularly scheduled visit before returning the patient to her bed. The ward clerk (who could communicate with all patients through the intercom) was instructed to respond in very specific ways. If the patient reported that she had fallen out of the bed, the clerk was instructed to inform the patient via the intercom that she would be assisted during her next scheduled visit and inform the patient how long it would be until that occurred. If the patient was merely screaming for assistance, the clerk informed her that the nursing staff had been there and reminded the patient to pick up the tongue depressors and count them to prove this to herself.

The hourly visits and the response of the nursing staff (including the use of the tongue depressors and the fact that she would be assisted only during regularly scheduled visits) were explained thoroughly to the patient. During the first day, she fell out of the bed about 10 minutes after a regularly scheduled nursing visit; she remained on the floor for 50 minutes until the next scheduled visit. Later that same day, she fell out of bed again, only this time it was about one-half hour after the last nursing visit; she remained on the floor for that half hour. Again on that same day she fell out of bed a third time; it was about 45 minutes after the last visit, and she remained on the floor for only 15 minutes. This was her last instance of falling out of bed, and by the third day, the restraints were removed. During the night of the first day, she called out for nursing assistance a couple of times; each time she was reminded to count the tongue depressors. By the second night, she no longer called out for assistance, because she was easily able to reassure herself that she had been visited regularly by counting the tongue depressors. Thus, within 2 or 3 days, all of the major "problems" had been resolved. Because she was no longer a cause of nursing staff anger, they were able to respond more appropriately to her and provide her with the psychosocial support she so desperately needed. In addition, because there was no need to take therapy time to discuss her "bad" behavior, that time could be spent dealing with the many issues related to Linda's illness. By taking a different approach with the patient to solve the problem, she quickly stopped screaming and stopped jumping out of bed. The nursing staff then became less angry at her and were more willing to provide her with the social support she needed to tolerate the various surgeries.

An important key factor in this case was convincing the staff that the intervention was not only appropriate but also virtually the only option. As you can imagine, it goes against everything a nurse is taught to ignore a patient who is calling out for assistance or to leave a patient who has fallen from the bed lying on the floor for as much as an hour. Talking the nurses into doing so was an extremely delicate task, and it raises yet another important issue in the possible barriers to communication—inflexibility on the part of therapists. Part of the stereotype of psychiatrists and psychologists is that they see a person for 50 minutes and 50 minutes only; regardless of what the patient may be talking about when the time is up, the session ends and the therapy is continued during the next session. The psychiatrist who had seen the patient came once each day for 50 minutes exactly. Holding fast to such a schedule would have prevented the intervention just described from even being considered. To convince nursing staff to ignore the patient, the therapist had to promise to be available to talk with staff or meet with them whenever the need arose; in actuality, the staff never called with an emergency request. The staff never needed to, because the therapist "dropped in" on the ward four or five times a day and phoned around 10 o'clock at night during each of the first few days of the intervention just to see how things were going and to listen to problems and concerns the staff were experiencing. This time was in addition to therapy time spent with the patient. This type of flexibility is extremely important in dealing with medical personnel. They perceive themselves as being available to patients at all hours of the day or night and see psychological services as rigid and unresponsive to the needs of patients; communication with them is improved if, in cases such as this when you need to provide support and encouragement to the staff, you make yourself available to staff on a flexible basis. Once you have communicated to medical personnel that you will go out of your way to help them cope with problems when they arise, you will have done much to remove many of the barriers to communication.

In summary then, a number of factors contribute to poor communication between therapists and medical specialists. First, many trained health professionals feel that mental health treatment consists primarily of listening and support, and thus they do not feel that another practitioner needs to become involved, given that everyone has those skills. Second, many health professionals do not see mental health services as being valuable or important because they have had bad experiences with traditional psychologists, psychiatrists, and other therapists who failed to solve the problem. Because medicine emphasizes immediate results, medical practitioners have little patience for the time that traditional psychotherapy approaches entail. Finally, many medical practitioners see psychiatrists and psychologists as inflexible and rigid, insisting on limiting their contact to 50 continuous minutes; making yourself available at unscheduled times to provide advice, support, or reassurance may help alleviate some of this.

Methods to Improve Communication

One of the best ways to facilitate the treatment of your patients is to develop relationships with medical specialists who are likely to refer to you and to whom you are likely to refer. Although the exact specialties you should consider are by necessity dictated by the nature of your practice, a number of specialties apply to virtually any therapist. These include neurology, endocrinology, obstetrics and gynecology (OB/GYN), internal medicine, and psychiatry. You should attempt to find a practitioner in *each specialty* with whom you can work and build a professional relationship.

One way to facilitate a relationship is to refer patients to physicians. Every patient you see should be asked if he or she has had a recent (in the past year) physical. Women patients in particular should be asked if they have had a recent OB/GYN examination with a PAP test and a thyroid panel. If patients have not had a physical, they should be strongly encouraged to have one. We have gone so far as to refuse to see patients who will not have a physical exam prior to beginning therapy. If a patient has her own doctor, you can obtain consent to communicate with that doctor, and you should encourage the woman to see her personal physician. If the woman does not have a physician of her own, you can refer the woman to one of the physicians on your list.

How to Make a Referral

Many nonmedical mental health professionals treat making physician referrals as a passive process. That is, they merely tell the patient to see a physician without assisting in making that happen and then wait for the results of the physical examination. This type of referral is rarely helpful either to the physician or to the mental health therapist; more active steps must be taken.

The major way you can assist in the referral process is by providing the physician with a few possible hypotheses about what may be going on with the patient. These hypotheses should be physical in nature, not, for example, theories about the patient's relationship with her family. In other words, if you wonder whether the depressive symptoms you are seeing might be the result of a thyroid disorder, say so when you make the referral. Physicians are taught to evaluate patients using what is called the "reasonable under the circumstances" definition of health, not the "optimal functioning" definition: Their goal is not to identify *any* possible symptom that may be interfering with optimal functioning. Rather, physicians are taught that, unless something is obviously abnormal, one should assume that the person is basically healthy. They are guided in these decisions by what the patient feels is bothering her and what she chooses to disclose. If the patient feels that her depression is the result of psychological factors (and she must have at some point or she would not be seeing you), she may not feel that these are relevant to disclose during the physical examination (as we saw in the case of Thelma in Chapter 2). Thus, in the absence of this information and without other clearly abnormal signs suggesting it be done, a physician may not order the thyroid panel necessary to determine if indeed the woman does have a thyroid condition. It is the responsibility of the mental health therapist to raise the issue and to direct the physician toward entertaining this diagnosis.

Many laypeople (mental health therapists included) are intimidated by the language of medicine. This is a serious problem for mental health practitioners who want to have mutually beneficial referral relationships with physicians. To solve this problem, it is necessary for nonmedical practitioners to learn at least some of the language of medicine. For example, if you routinely refer women for OB/GYN examinations, you need to know the difference between vaginismus and vaginitis. One (vaginismus, or involuntary tightening of the muscles around the vagina, often making intercourse painful or even impossible) is usually treated by a sex therapist, whereas the other (vaginitis, known commonly as a "yeast infection") is treated by a gynecologist. You do not have to *be* a physician; you merely need to be able to understand them when they talk to you. In addition, you need to be able to state your hypotheses in medical terms and to make specific requests for what evaluations you may need *in a language the physician can understand.* This includes using the term *patient.* Although many therapists have now discarded this term because they object to the underlying medical model it implies, when dealing with physicians, it is useful to call the women you are seeing *patients.* That is how physicians think of them, and if you want to facilitate communication, using language you do not necessarily agree with may be essential to this.

We have provided *some* of the necessary language in this book, but each mental health practitioner may need to know additional terms based on his or her unique practice. Nursing textbooks can often be extremely helpful in assisting nonmedical mental health practitioners in learning the language because of the careful, relatively nontechnical descriptions they use. The goal of nursing textbooks is not to allow nurses to diagnose and treat medical problems but, rather, to familiarize student nurses with the type of diseases and problems patients may face so that they are better able to work with physicians. If you routinely refer to certain medical specialists, obtain copies of *nursing textbooks for that specialty* and become familiar with the language in them. You will then be better able to communicate with physicians.

One additional matter: Do not pretend to understand something that you do not. When talking with a physician, do not merely smile and shake your head if he or she uses language with which you are unfamiliar. Assuming you have learned some of the basics of medical language, if an illness or diagnostic procedure is mentioned and you are not familiar with it, ask. No one expects you to know everything a physician knows. A physical problem affecting one of your patients may have serious implications for your therapy, and it is important to understand exactly what that problem (or procedure your patient will be undergoing) is. Most physicians will appreciate your interest in what they are doing. In addition, you can often be helpful in explaining the diagnosis or the upcoming medical procedure to the patient. However, to do so, *you* must understand what the diagnosis or the procedure is. Your goal is to make whatever you and the physician are doing for your patient a cooperative enterprise.

In addition to knowing the language, having some information to support your hypotheses is also useful when making a referral. Obtain data whenever possible. Thus, if you suspect hypothyroidism, ask your patient about weight fluctuations and attempts to gain or lose weight. Obtain some basic information about what your patient eats in a typical day and how that volume of food is related to weight changes. Ask about sleeping patterns and skin and hair changes. Making a referral to rule out hypothyroidism is easier if you can also say the woman has been dieting for about 4 months and that despite eating (by her report) less than 750 calories a day, she has not lost any weight. Do not expect the physician to obtain the same wealth of information you can obtain from your patient. The typical physician visit is *7 to 10 minutes long*. Presumably, you have met with your patient for at least 1 hour before you make the referral, and thus, you should have a lot of information that you can provide that would assist the physician in determining if the cause of the psychological presentation is indeed physical. If you are able to speak the language, have adequate data to support your hypotheses, and can relate the data to possible physical disorders, you will find that most physicians will readily do the evaluations and tests necessary to determine the nature of the possible physical problem.

Case Example: Rita

Rita, a patient who had been diagnosed with multiple sclerosis by her family physician, was referred for evaluation because of concerns about possible psychosomatic causes of her symptoms. The diagnosis of multiple sclerosis was in question because she did not have many of the typical signs (e.g., vision problems) of the disease (this was before the time that MRI was available to determine the presence of demyelinization). She had begun to lose motor function in all four extremities and had been confined to a wheelchair. Nursing staff and medical staff reported observing severe grand mal-type seizures in this patient, although repeated electroencephalograms (EEGs) were always normal. In interviews with her, she reported environmental events that she felt precipitated these seizures. Specifically, she felt she was most likely to have one when she was connected to an I-VAC machine (a device that controls the administration of intravenous medication). Some medications cannot be introduced continuously into a patient's veins; rather, a specified amount must be administered every few seconds or so to ensure that adequate dosage is obtained. The I-VAC machine makes a characteristic "beeping" noise when medicine is released. The patient felt that the sound of this beeping precipitated her seizures. Thus, to see what type of neurological changes accompanied her seizures, it was recommended to the neurologist that she receive an EEG evaluation with an I-VAC machine plugged in and running in the room. To convince the neurologist to do so, data on the number of previous EEGs performed that had revealed nothing, the number of witnessed seizures that the patient had had while in the hospital, and the number of times these seizures occurred while the patient was on an I-VAC machine were presented to the neurology staff. Despite the bizarreness of the request (typically, EEGs are not done with other, unnecessary equipment in the room), the data provided convinced the neurologist that it was worth a try. During the EEG with the I-VAC machine, the patient exhibited tonic-clonic convulsions consistent with a grand mal seizure and witnessed by a number of medical staff people; there was, however, *no evidence of abnormal discharges on the EEG.* Thus, the neurologist had clear evidence that these were pseudoseizures (psychiatric rather than neurological seizures), and treatment changed dramatically (for a complete description of this case, see Klonoff, Youngner, Moore, & Hershey, 1983-1984). From that point on, almost all of the neurology staff members were willing to agree to whatever recommendations for neurological testing the mental health staff members had, even if those recommendations were somewhat unconventional.

This case example demonstrates two points. First, with adequate data to support your hypotheses, you can make even unusual requests of physicians and they will likely agree and comply. Second, it underscores the importance of having a few successes to your future interactions with physicians. Once you have aided them in diagnosing a problem, they will be more willing to accept your recommendations in the future. You can do this, however, only if you make informed, data-based referrals with specific possible physical disorders in mind and with specific questions to be answered by the physician.

Maintaining Communication With Physicians

Regardless of whether you are referring your patient to a physician or he or she is referring a patient to you, keeping the physician informed of your progress is a necessary responsibility in maintaining good relationships with physicians. There are a number of factors to consider in keeping your medical colleagues informed.

Informed Consent

Of course, you cannot reveal any information you obtained or have any information revealed to you without first obtaining a release from your patient. *A release to speak with your patient's physician should be a routine part of your first-session office procedure.* Every patient you see, regardless of presenting problem or psychiatric diagnosis, should sign such a release, and you should routinely communicate with each patient's physician. You should not wait until you have reason to think a physical problem is present before you communicate with your patient's physician. This can be extremely distressing to patients; they will try to figure out exactly why all of a sudden you are talking to them about some type of physical problem. When you describe your need to share information with their physician as stemming from trying to ensure that *all* aspects of a patient are being cared for simultaneously, few patients will fail to give their consent.

However, from time to time, you will come across a patient who refuses to give her consent. This could mean any one of a number of things. First, the patient may not have a physician with whom she feels comfortable and whom she calls her own. If that is the case, you can assist her by providing her with a referral to one of the physicians on your list. Second, the patient may not be satisfied with the physician she is seeing. Assuming that she is not talking about dissatisfaction with a psychiatrist (with whom the strategy for dealing is different and will not be addressed here), the nature of her dissatisfaction needs to be identified. Does she find the physician's manner offensive or is she put off by him or her in some way (e.g., does she feel the physician is cold or uncaring)? Does she feel her physician does not listen to her or take sufficient time to really understand her problems? Is there some reason why your patient does not trust her physician? Or is the problem that your patient does not like the diagnoses (or lack of diagnoses) she has received? Sometimes, a patient's stated dissatisfaction with a physician is really dissatisfaction with the way her medical care is obtained (e.g., anger at her health maintenance organization [HMO], feeling as if she gets the runaround because she is on welfare, and so forth). It is important to help your patient sort through what is really dissatisfaction with a physician and what may be dissatisfaction for other reasons. Sometimes, patients misattribute the behaviors of physicians, and a therapist can be very helpful in clarifying alternative explanations. Similarly, sometimes patients (and therapists) do not realize how annoying or bothersome some patients can be, particularly patients who seem to call the physician all the time with no clear reason. The intervention of a therapist, who is making a referral with clear questions in mind, can often help improve a poor physician-patient relationship, thereby increasing the chance that your patient will get the medical attention she might need.

There are times, however, when it may be necessary to help your patient find a new physician. Your patient's prior relationship with her physician may be so tainted that any attempts to work with the physician may fail. Or you may have reason to believe that the physician is not doing a good job with your patient (i.e., you question the physician's competence). In those instances, it is helpful if you can refer your patient to one of the physicians on your list with whom you have had positive interactions in the past. Some physicians are more receptive than others to dealing with potentially "problem" patients, and it might be useful to have your patient seen by one of these. In addition, some physicians are more "psychologically minded"—that is, they are more comfortable dealing with emotional issues, patients, or both. These physicians may be willing to spend a little more time with your patient and may be more sensitive to potential stress-related signs and symptoms. Again, however, it is important that if you assist your patient in changing physicians, you remain active in the referral process.

Finally, sometimes despite your best efforts, a patient will still refuse to give her consent to allow you to communicate with her physician. We feel strongly that continuing to see the patient under these circumstances is a mistake. Assuming that you have explained that the purpose of the communication is to ensure that all aspects of the patient are appropriately attended to, the continued refusal is a serious red flag to your work with the patient. What might the patient be hiding? Why does she maintain her refusal? Perhaps the patient feels that her physician will give you information that may be somehow damaging to her. If this is the case, you should take sufficient time with your patient so that she understands that you will be making your own independent judgment about her and her problems and that the information from her physician will only supplement these, not supplant them. Sometimes, the patient does not want her physician to know she is seeing you for some reason. Her physician may be a family friend, or she may just not want anyone to know that she is experiencing psychological problems. Again, it is important to explain to the patient that you would be doing her a disservice to not communicate with her physician. For her physician to provide her with optimal medical care, he or she needs to know about all of the problems the patient might be having, not merely those in which the patient thinks the doctor might be interested. All of these questions and issues must be addressed before therapy can progress. We have gone so far as to make consent to communicate with a patient's physician a condition of continuing in therapy.

What to Communicate

Although, for you, the satisfaction of doing therapy may be trying to figure out, for example, the relationship between childhood experiences and the current presenting symptoms or unraveling the associations between the maladaptive behavior and the reinforcers for that behavior, it is unlikely that your patients' physicians derive the same enjoyment from this information. (If they did, wouldn't they have chosen psychiatry as a specialty?) Long theoretical discussions of your hypotheses regarding how and why the patient is experiencing the current symptoms and problems are unnecessary in communications with physicians and will turn them off; save them for your colleagues or psychiatry grand rounds. Physicians view patients whom they refer for mental health services as "problems" who have not responded to the standard physical interventions, so they need to be dealt with by someone else. Thus, they are primarily interested in the degree to which the problem is being solved—that is, in the progress being made. Typically, they do not care *how* that progress is made, just as long as it is. Therefore, you do not need to include complicated psychological conceptualizations in your report to physicians. Rather, you will need to indicate what information you are using to evaluate patient progress, say how this information is obtained, and offer an assessment of the patient's progress to date. You should also include your future treatment plans with the patient.

How to Communicate

It is important to communicate with physicians in a manner that they are likely to understand. A number of medical fields learned to keep patient notes and chart patient progress using what has come to be called the "SOAP" format. SOAP stands for (a) S = subjective, or what the patient describes the problem to be, often quoted as the patient's own words; (b) O = objective, or the evaluator's description of the presenting problem, including a description of the physical examination performed, the various tests prescribed, and the results of the physical examination and the tests; (c) A = assessment, or an overall evaluation of what the results of the various diagnostic indicators suggest the patient's problem is; and (d) P = plan, a description of what the physician intends to do to ameliorate the problem. Although you do not have to use this format exactly, you need to be aware that *this is the type of information a physician is looking for in your communication with him or her.* Most crucial in this type of communication is the plan. When providing information to a physician, it is important to describe *exactly what* you intend to do, *how* you intend to do it, and *when* it will be completed. As described earlier, one of the things that gives mental health professionals a bad reputation with physicians is the notion that patients embarking on a course of psychotherapy are beginning an undefined, indefinite process with no clear criteria for success and no reasonable estimate of the time it will take. By contrast, if a physician prescribes a 10-day course of antibiotics, he or she knows that by the end of the 10-day period, either the patient will be "cured" or a different diagnosis, treatment, or both will need to be considered.

To work effectively with physicians, *your treatment plan needs to be sufficiently clear and needs to entail a reasonable course of treatment.* Even if you foresee therapy taking a number of months, you should build into your treatment plan *periodic reevaluations,* including criteria for improvement, so that you can recommunicate with the referring physician regarding your patient's progress. If for some reason you are unable to meet the time frame you originally anticipated, you should communicate that (and the reasons why your original estimates proved to be incorrect) to the referring physician so that he or she will still feel informed about the patient's progress. This type of communication often has additional side benefits for you. Systematically thinking through the progress you have made with a patient and identifying your specific plans for future work with her can help you focus your treatment and ensure that you are providing the best care possible.

Summary

One of the most important things you can do for your patient is to work cooperatively with her physician. This is true regardless of whether the problem is primarily psychological or primarily physical. Communication with *every* patient's medical doctor should be a routine part of your practice to ensure that all possible causes of your patient's distress are being adequately considered. Despite the inherent barriers to communication between physicians and therapists, it is your responsibility to establish and maintain communication. Every patient you see should be required to have had a physical examination within the past 6 months to 1 year. If not, the patient should schedule one concurrent with your treatment. When you refer a patient for a medical evaluation, you should be an active participant in that evaluation, providing possible hypotheses about what may be wrong and, when indicated, providing data to support those hypotheses. You should become familiar with the medical terminology, common diseases, and diagnostic procedures that are most relevant to your practice so that you can communicate with physicians in an informed manner. You should make yourself available to discuss questions or concerns medical personnel might have about your patient and the nature of her treatment. You need to become comfortable with briefly describing what your treatment will be, the intended outcome of your treatment, the criteria you will use to determine whether your treatment is successful, and the time frame in which your treatment will occur. You can expect that your physician colleague will do the same. Only when mental health and physical health are considered simultaneously can misdiagnoses be prevented.

Reference

Klonoff, E. A., Youngner, S. A., Moore, D. J., & Hershey, L. (1983-1984). Chronic factitious illness: A behavioral approach. *International Journal of Psychiatry in Medicine, 13*(3), 173-183.

11

Conclusions

Throughout this book, we have emphasized that physical disorders can be (and often are) misdiagnosed as psychiatric and that this misdiagnosis always entails a misattribution about the nature and cause of apparently psychiatric symptoms. The attributional error that leads to the misdiagnosis can come from the patient or her therapist. For example, Thelma (Chapter 2) attributed her physical symptoms to her thyroid disorder but her associated depression to psychiatric causes, so her physical disorder was never adequately treated. In the case of Miriam (Chapter 8), the patient herself misattributed her experience of rapid heartbeat to anxiety and then misattributed her "anxiety" to various environmental stimuli, which then led to the development of agoraphobia. Likewise, Jackie (Chapter 6) misattributed her symptoms of focal sensory seizures to her dead mother, therapists misattributed that claim to a delusion, and the misdiagnosis of schizophrenia was the outcome. Mindy (Chapter 7) similarly misattributed her primictal event (hallucinations of groups of voices) to being a medium who could communicate with the dead, her husband misattributed this to psychopathology on her part, and mental health professionals agreed with him. Numerous therapists misattributed the many symptoms presented by Kate (described in detail in the Introduction) to a diversity of psychiatric disorders. Misdiagnosis of physical disorders as psychiatric thus entails the tendency of laypeople and clinicians alike to assume that everything and anything—from obvious family factors to paranormal entities—*except a physical disorder* is the explanation for psychiatric symptoms.

By emphasizing the serious and even lethal consequences of such misattributions, we hope to make therapists more aware of them. Making causal attributions—finding explanations—is a routine, instantaneous, and nearly unconscious aspect of ordinary cognition and, hence, of clinical cognition as well. For therapists, these attributions can no longer remain simple, automatic, reflexlike responses to apparently psychiatric symptoms; immediately attributing these symptoms to psychiatric causes must not continue. Because their consequences can range from serious to lethal, therapists' causal attributions about a patient's ostensibly psychiatric symptoms must become conscious, careful, data-based, deliberate decisions in which the therapist has carefully differentiated between the content (description) of a symptom (e.g., depression, anxiety) and the nature and cause of it. In the final analysis, therapists must begin to view themselves as more than people who treat psychological and behavioral problems, because in a sense, doing therapy is the lesser of the two things that therapists do. They must also begin to view themselves as people who—first and foremost—make causal attributions about those problems, which then determine the nature and course of treatment (and invariably of women's lives), thereby rendering such attributions the more significant of a therapist's two activities. For each woman being seen in therapy, each therapist must ask himself or herself these questions: "What causal attributions have I made about her symptoms?" "Am I sure that I am right?" If the therapist's answer to the latter question is negative, it is the therapist's responsibility to take all necessary steps—including acquiring psychological, medical, and neurological tests—to make that answer affirmative, to safeguard, improve, and save the lives of women and girls.

In this book, we have focused only on *physical disorders whose psychiatric presentation leads them to be misdiagnosed as psychiatric disorders*. We have ignored other physical disorders that entail psychiatric symptoms, because these disorders are unlikely to be so misdiagnosed. For example, it is well-known that chronic obstructive pulmonary disease (Klonoff, Greene, Polefrone, Dambrocia, & Nochomovitz, 1986), sarcoidosis (Klonoff & Kleinhenz, 1993), and other physical disorders often involve, in addition to clear physical symptoms, signs of anxiety or panic attacks and that, similarly, diabetes often involves many psychiatric and neuropsychiatric symptoms above and beyond its physical presentation. These and other similar physical disorders, however, are unlikely to be misdiagnosed as psychiatric disorders because the primary, major clinical picture is unambiguously physical—which is not the case for the disorders detailed in this book. Likewise, we have ignored the many physical disorders for which psychiatric symptoms are often secondary and reactive; patients diagnosed with cancer or with certain chronic, neurological conditions often respond to their diagnosis with severe anxiety and depression that meet the clinical criteria for a psychiatric diagnosis and therefore demand therapeutic attention. Again, however, in both cases, *the physical disorder has been accurately diagnosed,* and the psychiatric symptoms are either a minor part of the symptom picture or a secondary part, appearing later; the physical disorder is not, and is extremely unlikely to be, misdiagnosed as psychopathology. For the disorders in this book, on the other hand, the major symptom picture of the physical disorder is psychiatric, and the disorder is likely to be misdiagnosed as such. Readers interested in the former types of disorders—diagnosed physical conditions with psychiatric complications—can consult any of the major textbooks in health psychology and behavioral medicine about the management of such cases and about the important role that therapists play in that.

In a nutshell, the message of this book is that many women who exhibit apparently psychiatric symptoms do not have psychiatric disorders but instead have underlying, undiagnosed physical disorders, and that these misdiagnosed physical problems in part may account for women's high rate (relative to men) of certain (ostensibly) psychiatric disorders. Do we mean to suggest by this that women are not "crazier" than men but are instead simply sicker, that women are not more prone to psychopathology but are instead more prone to physical illness because they are weak and sickly? No, we do not. There are many physical disorders that men tend to exhibit far more frequently than women, and many of these are lethal, serious disorders that play a role in men's higher mortality rate and shorter life span than women's; although women exhibit more frequent mild and acute physical problems, men exhibit more lethal physical problems such that neither sex could be described as "sicker" than the other (Klonoff & Landrine, 1992). Most of the physical disorders that are more common among men than women, however, *do not* manifest themselves in emotional and behavioral symptoms and hence are unlikely to be misdiagnosed as psychopathology. It is not that women are crazier or more sickly than men but, rather, that women tend to exhibit physical disorders whose symptom complexity has a higher probability of psychiatric misdiagnosis than do those of men.

Throughout this book, we have stated explicitly, implied, and presented cases illustrating that therapists are likely to misdiagnose the physical disorders described here as psychopathology. Do we mean to suggest by this that psychologists, counselors, and social workers are alone in such errors and that psychiatrists (therapists with medical backgrounds) do not make them; do we mean to suggest that nonmedical therapists therefore have no business doing treatment because their lack of medical training makes them dangerous in the ways detailed here? No, we do not. In our collective clinical experience, the diagnostic and attributional errors detailed in this book have been made, and are made, irrespective of therapists' educational backgrounds and of the presence or absence of medical training. Our experiences are supported by the empirical evidence on the frequency of misdiagnosis presented at the start of this book (as well as throughout the references to the chapters) insofar as each of those studies examined the tendency *of psychiatrists* to misdiagnose physical disorders as psychiatric. Unfortunately, there is something about the presenting symptom of depression with suicidal ideation, for example, that leads all of us, regardless of training, to make one kind of diagnostic attribution rather than another and to draw conclusions rather than to continue to ask important questions about the causes of that symptom. Perhaps it is that our training as therapists (medical or not) has oversensitized us to psychopathology—has led us to search for it and subsequently perhaps to find it where it does not exist. In any event, because we all, whatever our clinical training, make these diagnostic errors, the information in this book should not be used in the battle between medicine and the other clinical sciences to disenfranchise some professionals, privilege others, and widen the gulf between professional, clinical camps. Instead, we suggest that the information here implies the need to narrow the gulf between disciplines and to forge new, cooperative relationships between professionals in social work, psychology, endocrinology, neurology, and other fields to improve the efficiency and quality of diagnosis and treatment. An underlying theme running throughout this book is the urgent need for consultation and cooperation among professionals to improve the outcome of clinical interventions for women, girls, and their therapists alike.

References

Klonoff, E. A., Greene, P., Polefrone, J., Dambrocia, J. P., & Nochomovitz, M. L. (1986, November). *Treatment of panic attacks associated with chronic obstructive pulmonary disease (COPD)*. Paper presented at the annual convention of the Association for Advancement of Behavior Therapy, Chicago.

Klonoff, E. A., & Kleinhenz, M. E. (1993). Psychological factors in sarcoidosis: The relationship between life stress and pulmonary function. *Sarcoidosis, 10,* 118-124.

Klonoff, E. A., & Landrine, H. (1992). Sex roles, occupational roles, and symptom-reporting: A test of competing hypotheses on sex differences. *Journal of Behavioral Medicine, 15*(4), 355-364.

Appendix A

The Relationship Between Various Psychiatric Disorders and Physical Disorders to Be Considered

| | Possible Physical Disorders to Consider | | |
Psychiatric Disorder	Endocrinological Disorder	Neurological Disorder	Other Disorder
Depressive disorders/dysthymia	Hyperthyroidism Hypothyroidism Addison's disease Cushing's syndrome Hypopituitarism Hypoparathyroidism/hypocalcemia (children) Hyperparathyroidism/hypercalcemia	Temporal lobe epilepsy [TLE] (prodromal and interictal stages) Multiple sclerosis	Lupus Wilson's disease Mitral valve prolapse
Bipolar disorders/cyclothymia	Hyperthyroidism Hypothyroidism Cushing's syndrome (with exogenous steroids)	Temporal lobe epilepsy (interictal stage) Multiple sclerosis	
Generalized anxiety disorder	Hyperthyroidism Hypoparathyroidism/hypocalcemia (children) Hyperparathyroidism/hypercalcemia Hypoglycemia	Auditory sensory seizures	Mitral valve prolapse Posterolateral sclerosis
Panic disorder/agoraphobia			Mitral valve prolapse
Obsessive/compulsive disorder		Temporal lobe epilepsy (interictal stage and paliacousia)	

Disorder	Endocrine/Metabolic	Seizure/Neurological	Autoimmune/Other
Somatization disorder	Hyperparathyroidism/hypercalcemia	Vertiginous sensory seizures Olfactory/gustatory hallucinations/seizures	Lupus Multiple sclerosis
Conversion disorder		Vertiginous sensory seizures Visual sensory seizures Auditory sensory seizures Olfactory/gustatory hallucinations/seizures	Lupus Posterolateral sclerosis Multiple sclerosis
Hypochondriasis	Hyperparathyroidism/hypercalcemia		Lupus Multiple sclerosis
Dissociative disorders		Temporal lobe epilepsy (aura and poriomania)	
Paraphilias		Temporal lobe epilepsy	
Eating disorders	Hypopituitarism		Lupus
Intermittent explosive disorder		Temporal lobe epilepsy	Lupus
Schizophrenia/other psychotic disorders	Hypothyroidism Cushing's syndrome Hypopituitarism	Somatosensory seizures Complex auditory hallucinations of TLE (interictal stage and if untreated for a number of years)	Lupus Wilson's disease Multiple sclerosis
Delirium/dementia	Hypothyroidism	Temporal lobe epilepsy (interictal stage)	Multiple sclerosis
Personality disorders	Hypopituitarism Hyperparathyroidism/hypercalcemia	Temporal lobe epilepsy (interictal stage)	Multiple sclerosis

Appendix B

*Questions to Ask Patients to Rule Out
Physical Disorders and Quick Symptom Guide*

Here, we present a cookbook summary of the questions (detailed in previous chapters) to include in an interview to distinguish psychiatric from organic disorders.

Major Symptom: Depression

1. *To rule out lupus:* Ask about presence of episodic joint and muscle pain; cough; fever; migraine headaches; arthritis; and chest and/or heart pain, along with nausea and morning stiffness, hypertension, anemia, and hepatitis; skin rash; history of taking or is currently taking thorazine, antihypertensive drugs, carbamazepine (Tegretol), antibiotics such as penicillin and streptomycin, succinimides such as Milontin and Zarontin, and other anticonvulsants such as Dilantin (phenytoin). Send for a physical.

2. *To rule out hyperthyroidism:* Ask about attacks of diarrhea, sweating, and generalized weakness; increased appetite *but with a loss of weight or stable weight;* red, puffy eyelids; history of depression in female relatives; history of frequent viral infections; sensation of a lump in the throat or of being strangled. Ask about most recent physical exam and recommend a physical with a thyroid panel.

3. *To rule out hypothyroidism:* Ask about fatigue, tiredness, and weakness; always feeling cold; tingling and numbness in the fingers (peripheral neuropathy); headaches; not hearing well; loss of appetite but *with weight gain;* constipation; stiff and aching muscles; and excessive and irregular menstrual bleeding. Observe for puffy red eyes and brittle hair that falls out. Ask about most recent physical exam and recommend a physical with a thyroid panel. On psychological tests, look for low scores on the Wechsler Adult Intelligence Scale (WAIS)

Digit Span, Vocabulary, and Block Design and impaired scores on the Halstead-Reitan Trailmaking Test. On the Minnesota Multiphasic Personality Inventory (MMPI), look for a pattern of clinically significant elevations on Scales 2, 6, 7, and 8 and also for all scores on all of the other subscales of the MMPI elevated in the T = 60 to 65 range.

4. *To rule out multiple sclerosis:* Ask about where she was born (check to see if it was north of Boulder, Colorado). Look for a low Similarities score on the WAIS. Ask about presence of ataxia, weakness, numbness and tingling sensations, and urinary incontinence in general. Assess whether psychiatric and other symptoms are increased under stress, when dehydrated (due to alcohol consumption or exercise), and in the presence of heat. Run the hot bath test. If positive, suggest that she have a nuclear magnetic resonance (NMR) test and a physical.

5. *To rule out Wilson's disease:* Ask about and observe for symptoms and signs of liver damage, such as cirrhosis and jaundice (swollen liver, whites of the eyes are yellow). Send for a physical.

6. *To rule out cancer of the pancreas:* Must be at least aged 50. If so, ask about abdominal pain and sense of impending doom. Send for a physical.

7. *To rule out Addison's disease:* Ask about craving for salt, increased salt intake, nausea, and vomiting. Send to an endocrinologist for an exam.

8. *To rule out Cushing's syndrome:* Ask about weight gain, hypertension, and amenorrhea (loss of menstrual periods), and observe for facial obesity—but none of these may be present. Send to an endocrinologist for an exam.

9. If a girl or teenage female rather than an adult, *to rule out hypoparathyroidism (hypocalcemia):* Ask about and observe for tingling and numbness in the face and hands; frequent headaches; seizures with convulsions; poor tooth development; childhood mental retardation; thin, patchy hair; muscular weakness; and painful cramplike spasms in the hands, feet, and throat (called *tetany*). Send to an endocrinologist for an exam.

10. *To rule out hyperparathyroidism (hypercalcemia) in adults:* Ask about dull back pain; frequent urinary tract infections; gastrointestinal dysfunctions, including nausea, vomiting, and constipation; and abdominal pain. Send to an endocrinologist for an exam.

11. *To rule out temporal lobe epilepsy:* Ask the general history questions given at the end of this appendix. Send to a psychologist or neuropsychologist for preliminary testing. If the tests and symptom patterns suggest complex partial seizures (CPS), send to a neurologist for an EEG.

Major Symptom: Anxiety

1. *To rule out mitral valve prolapse:* Ask about prior history of cardiac problems (has she ever been told that she had a benign heart murmur or that there were extra heart sounds). Send for an echocardiogram.

2. *To rule out hyperthyroidism:* Ask about attacks of diarrhea, sweating, and generalized weakness; increased appetite *but with a loss of weight or stable weight;* red, puffy eyelids; history of depression in female relatives; history of frequent viral infections; sensation of a lump in the throat or of being strangled. Ask about most recent physical exam and recommend a physical with a thyroid panel.

3. *To rule out multiple sclerosis:* Ask about where she was born (check to see if it was north of Boulder, Colorado). Look for a low Similarities score on the WAIS. Ask about presence of ataxia, weakness, numbness and tingling sensations, and urinary incontinence in general. Assess whether psychiatric and other symptoms are increased under stress, when dehydrated (due to alcohol consumption or exercise), and in the presence of heat. Run the hot bath test. If positive, suggest that she have an NMR and a physical.

4. *To rule out Wilson's disease:* Ask about and observe for symptoms and signs of liver damage, such as cirrhosis and jaundice (swollen liver, whites of the eyes are yellow). Send for a physical.

5. If a girl or teenage female rather than an adult, *to rule out hypoparathyroidism (hypocalcemia):* Ask about and observe for tingling and numbness in the face and hands; frequent headaches; seizures with convulsions; poor tooth development; childhood mental retardation; thin, patchy hair; muscular weakness; and painful cramplike spasms in the hands, feet, and throat (called *tetany*). Send to an endocrinologist for an exam.

6. *To rule out hyperparathyroidism (hypercalcemia) in adults:* Ask about dull back pain; frequent urinary tract infections; gastrointestinal dysfunctions, including nausea, vomiting, and constipation; and abdominal pain. Send to an endocrinologist for an exam.

7. *To rule out temporal lobe epilepsy:* Ask the general history questions given at the end of this appendix. Send to a psychologist or neuropsychologist for preliminary testing. If the tests and symptom patterns suggest CPS, send to a neurologist for an EEG.

Major Symptom: Bipolar Disorder

1. *To rule out hyperthyroidism:* Ask about attacks of diarrhea, sweating, and generalized weakness; increased appetite *but with a loss of weight or stable weight;* red, puffy eyelids; history of depression in female relatives; history of frequent viral infections; sensation of a lump in the throat or of being strangled. Ask about most recent physical exam and recommend a physical with a thyroid panel.

2. *To rule out temporal lobe epilepsy:* Ask the general history questions given at the end of this appendix. Send to a psychologist or neuropsychologist for preliminary testing. If the tests and symptom patterns suggest CPS, send to a neurologist for an EEG.

Major Symptom: Personality Disorder

Histrionic or dependent personality with or without somatization:

1. *To rule out multiple sclerosis:* Ask about where she was born (check to see if it was north of Boulder, Colorado). Look for a low Similarities score on the WAIS. Ask about presence of ataxia, weakness, numbness and tingling sensations, and urinary incontinence in general. Assess whether psychiatric and other symptoms are increased under stress, when dehydrated (due to alcohol consumption or exercise), and in the presence of heat. Run the hot bath test. If positive, suggest that she have an NMR.

2. *To rule out Wilson's disease:* Ask about and observe for symptoms and signs of liver damage, such as cirrhosis and jaundice (swollen liver, whites of the eyes are yellow). Send for a physical.

3. If a girl or teenage female rather than an adult, *to rule out hypoparathyroidism (hypocalcemia):* Ask about and observe for tingling and numbness in the face and hands; frequent headaches; seizures with convulsions; poor tooth development; childhood mental retardation; thin, patchy hair; muscular weakness, and painful cramplike spasms in the hands, feet, and throat (called *tetany*). Send to an endocrinologist for an exam.

4. *To rule out hyperparathyroidism (hypercalcemia) in adults:* Ask about dull back pain; frequent urinary tract infections; gastrointestinal dysfunctions, including nausea, vomiting, and constipation; and abdominal pain. Send to an endocrinologist for an exam.

5. *To rule out temporal lobe epilepsy:* Ask the general history questions given at the end of this appendix. Send to a psychologist or neuropsychologist for preliminary testing. If the tests and symptom patterns suggest CPS, send to a neurologist for an EEG.

Other Symptoms

For symptoms of schizophrenia, lost time, multiple personality disorder, fugue, episodic dyscontrol, schizotypal personality, and sexual deviance consider possible CPS.

Questions to Ask to Assess for Possible CPS

To evaluate for possible CPS, it is important to know about the presence or absence of the following, early childhood risk factors through careful interview:

1. Head trauma in infancy or childhood
2. Prolonged, high fevers in infancy

3. Low birth weight
4. Loss of consciousness during childhood
5. Maintained in incubator as an infant
6. Infantile seizures were present
7. Complications in the delivery of the patient (e.g., a forceps delivery, an unusually long labor, muconeum staining)
8. School performance, particularly signs of learning disability (failure in one subject, such as math or reading) and being left back a grade
9. The extent to which the patient met early childhood developmental norms on time such as sitting up, crawling, walking, and talking on time
10. Anoxia at birth
11. Significant drug and alcohol use by the mother when pregnant with the patient
12. Significant smoking by the mother when pregnant with the patient

The presence of any of the following current factors is also suggestive:

1. Presence of a vascular disease
2. History of constant or frequent infectious diseases
3. Presence of hypoglycemia or other disorders of glucose metabolism
4. Poisoning (by lead, arsenic, etc.) at any time
5. Current and previous alcohol and drug use or abuse

In the end, the patient's symptom pattern should alert the therapist to the possibility of CPS, that pattern presented in detail in Chapter 6. *If the patient's symptoms are consistent with CPS,* the presence of any three early childhood risk factors is sufficient to entertain CPS as a possibility and the referral procedures outlined here should be initiated. If more than three of the early childhood factors are present and the patient's symptoms are consistent with CPS, the possibility of CPS may be considered good and the referral procedures outlined earlier for CPS should be followed.

Glossary

a Prefix meaning *without*.

Addison's disease A disorder caused by a deficiency of the corticosteroids produced by the adrenal cortex.

Adversive seizures This type of elementary focal seizure occurs in the premotor area of the frontal lobe and is characterized by a deviation of the head, eyes, and body to the opposite side of the seizure focus.

Agnosia An inability to recognize objects despite adequate information about them reaching the brain via the sense organs. It is usually associated with a specific sense, such as tactile, visual, or auditory agnosia, in which the patient is unable to recognize objects by touch, sight, or hearing, respectively.

Agraphia Loss of or reduced ability to write despite normal function of hands and arm muscles.

Akasthesia An inability to sit still, often seen as a side effect of antipsychotic medication but also seen in patients with Parkinson's disease.

Akinesia Complete or almost complete loss of movement, particularly of the ability to initiate movement.

Alexia The inability to recognize and name written words.

Amenorrhea The absence of menstrual periods.

Amygdala One of the structures in the limbic system of the brain, the amygdala is involved in the control of some emotional responses.

Anhedonia The inability to experience pleasure.

Anomia The inability to name things.

Anoxia The absence of oxygen within brain tissue. *Hypoxia* is the reduction of oxygen supply to a body area.

Anterior Related to the front of the body. In humans, this is synonymous with *ventral*.

Apathetic thyrotoxicosis A form of hyperthyroidism that occurs in the aged, characterized by severe depression with extreme apathy and withdrawal.

Aphasia   A disturbance of previously acquired language caused by some type of cerebral dysfunction. Aphasia can affect the ability to speak, write, comprehend, and/or read language.

Asomatognosis   The inability to recognize one's body as one's own.

Astereognosis   The inability to recognize objects by touch when they are placed in one hand.

Ataxia   Lack of coordination and clumsiness. This may affect balance and gait, limb or eye movements, and/or speech.

Atonic seizures   Seizures characterized by loss of muscle tension.

Auditory sensory seizure   This type of seizure has a focus in the superior temporal gyrus and is characterized by hearing buzzing, ringing, and hissing sounds.

Aura   The warning sensation that precedes or marks the onset of a seizure or a migraine headache. For persons with seizures, the aura may consist of distorted perception (such as a hallucinatory sound or smell) or a sensation of movement in the body.

Auscultation   The procedure of listening to sounds within the heart, using a stethoscope, to detect the presence of disease.

Autoimmune disorder   Any of numerous disorders caused by a reaction of the person's immune system against the organs and tissues of his or her own body.

Automatism   A state in which an individual carries out movements and activities without being aware of doing so and with no memory later of what happened. The episodes usually last only a few minutes.

Basal ganglia   Nerve cell clusters in the cerebrum and brain stem that play a role in producing smooth, continuous muscle actions and in stopping and starting movements.

Benign heart murmur   An extra heart sound heard during auscultation that is not considered dangerous or needing treatment. It is often found in patients with mitral valve prolapse.

Bilateral   Affecting both sides of the body or both organs if they are paired (e.g., both eyes in bilateral paralysis).

Carbohydrates   A group of substances that (along with fat) provide the body with energy. An essential ingredient of a healthy diet, sugar and starch are probably the most familiar of these substances.

Caudate Nucleus   A structure in the brain that is part of the basal ganglia, the portion of the brain that is involved in control of the body's motor tone and gross intentional movements.

Central nervous system (CNS)   The brain and the spinal cord.

Cerebellum   A rounded structure located behind the brain stem concerned primarily with maintenance of posture and balance and coordination of movement.

Cingulate gyrus   One of the cortical structures in the limbic system.

Circumstantiality   A characteristic of speech in which the speaker provides incidental information that is full of details but not of primary importance to the topic at hand.

Clonic phase   Part of a grand mal seizure during which there is generalized, bilateral severe convulsions of the body and limbs.

Clonic seizures   Seizures characterized by rhythmical contractions of the muscles.

Complex auditory hallucination Hearing music or words as a result of focal seizure activity.

Complex visual illusions These entail perceived changes of three-dimensional visual space and are most commonly associated with seizures in the right hemisphere temporo-occipital region.

contra- Prefix meaning *contrary* or *opposite.*

Contralateral On the opposite side.

Corpus callosum The broad band of neural fibers that joins the two sides of the brain, sending information from one side to the other.

Corticosteroids A group of hormones produced by the adrenal glands that control the use of nutrients and the excretion of salts and water in the urine.

Cushing's syndrome A disorder caused by an abnormally high level of circulating corticosteroid hormones, which are produced naturally by the adrenal glands.

Diabetes mellitus A disorder in which the pancreas produces insufficient or no insulin, the hormone responsible for the absorption of glucose into the cells to meet their energy needs. As a result, the level of glucose in the blood becomes abnormally high, causing increased urination, thirst, and hunger. Weight loss, fatigue, and accelerated degeneration of small blood vessels result.

Diastole The resting period of the heart muscle.

dys- A prefix meaning *abnormal, difficult, painful,* or *faulty.*

Dystonia Abnormal muscle rigidity resulting in painful muscle spasms, oddly fixed postures, or strange movement patterns. Although most dystonia is the result of neurological disease, it may also be a side effect of antipsychotic medication (dystonic reactions).

Echocardiography A method of obtaining an image of the heart structure using ultrasound, which is reflected differently by each part of the heart, resulting in a complex series of echoes.

EEG Electroencephalogram, a procedure that records the minute electrical impulses produced by the brain. Because some seizures occur only when the brain is stressed, EEGs may be done after the person has been sleep deprived for a period of time (sleep-deprived EEG), while the person is hyperventilating, or while the person is looking at a flashing light (EEG with photic driving).

Elementary auditory hallucination The perception of nonexistent environmental stimuli as a result of seizure activity. A common feature of all elementary auditory hallucinations is that the patient recognizes them as pathological (as opposed to someone with schizophrenia, for whom the hallucinations are not seen as abnormal).

Elementary auditory illusion Misperceptions of actual environmental stimuli as a result of seizure activity. Sounds are heard as louder than normal, softer than normal, or as increasing or decreasing in rhythm or tone.

Elementary visual illusion Changes in the perceptual quality of an object. These can include changes in perceived size, dimensions of an object, color, movement, and pace of movement of an object. These often occur as primictal events.

Endocrine glands Glands that secrete chemicals, called hormones, directly into the bloodstream (that is, not through a duct) to be transported to organs and tissues throughout the body.

Endogenous Arising from causes within the body.

Epidemiology The study of the rates of disease among groups of people by age, gender, ethnicity, etc.

Epilepsy A disease characterized by recurrent seizures or temporary alterations in one or more brain functions.

Epinephrine A naturally occurring hormone (also called adrenaline) that is one of two chemicals released by the adrenal gland in response to signals from the sympathetic division of the autonomic nervous system. The signals are triggered by stress, exercise, and emotions such as fear.

Etiology Cause, origin.

Exocrine glands Glands that secrete substances through a duct onto the inner surface of an organ or onto the outer surface of the body. Examples include salivary glands, which release saliva into the mouth; lacrimal glands, which release tears; and sweat glands.

Exogenous Arising from causes outside of the body, such as external infections, poisoning, or injury.

Extrapyramidal nervous system A network of nerve pathways linking nuclei in the cerebrum, the basil ganglia, and parts of the brain stem that influences and modifies the electrical impulses sent from the brain to the skeletal muscles. Damage to this system can cause disturbances in voluntary (willed) movements and in muscle tone, as well as the appearance of involuntary movements, such as tremors, jerking, or writhing movements. Damage can be the result of various diseases as well as a side effect of taking phenothiazine medications.

Fissures Deep furrows or grooves in the brain that divide each hemisphere into distinct areas known as the frontal, parietal, temporal, and occipital lobes.

Focal motor seizure This type of elementary partial seizure begins in the frontal cortex and involves tonic-clonic movements on the opposite side of the body.

Focal seizures Seizures that occur in only a small, focused portion of the brain.

Global hyposexuality One of the symptoms of temporal lobe epilepsy (complex partial seizures). The patient has a chronic, global absence of sexual desires, an absence of an interest in sex, and rarely experiences genital arousal.

Globus pallidus One of the structures in the brain that comprises the basal ganglia.

Glucose The body's chief source of energy for cell metabolism. Its major source is from the digestion of carbohydrates.

Glucose tolerance test This test provides more complete information about the presence of a disturbance in carbohydrate metabolism. The patient receives a predetermined amount of glucose orally, and plasma glucose levels are then measured fasting and at half-hour or 1-hour intervals.

-gnosia Suffix meaning *recognition of.*

Grand mal seizures Seizures in which the person falls to the ground unconscious and suffers generalized jerky muscle contractions. Although the seizure itself may last for only a few minutes, the person usually remains unconscious for a time and may have no recall of the seizure after awakening. Some people experience an aura prior to the actual seizure.

-graphia A suffix meaning *writing.*

Graves' disease An autoimmune disorder characterized by an overactive thyroid gland resulting in excessive production of thyroid hormones.

Gustatory Having to do with the sense of taste.

Gustatory hallucination   The fleeting perception of a strange taste that is a primictal event.

hemi-   Prefix meaning *half.*

Hepatolenticular degeneration   See **Wilson's disease.**

Hippocampal gyrus   One of the brain structures that compose the limbic system.

Hippocampus   One of the brain structures that compose the limbic system.

Homeostasis   The dynamic processes used by an organism to maintain a constant internal environment despite external changes.

Hyperethicality   High or excess moralism.

Hyperglycemia   An abnormally high level of glucose in the blood, typically associated with untreated or poorly controlled diabetes mellitus.

Hypergraphia   High level of or excessive writing.

Hyperparathyroidism   Overactivity of the parathyroid glands, which results in increased levels of calcium in the blood (hypercalcemia).

Hypersomnia   Abnormally high amount of time spent sleeping.

Hypertension   Abnormally high blood pressure, usually defined as a resting blood pressure greater than 140 mm Hg (systolic)/90 mm Hg (diastolic).

Hyperthyroidism   Overactivity of the thyroid glands, resulting in overproduction of thyroid hormones.

Hypoglycemia   An abnormally low level of glucose in the blood.

Hypoparathyroidism   Insufficient production of parathyroid hormone by the parathyroid glands, resulting in low levels of calcium in the blood and tissue fluids (hypocalcemia).

Hypothalamus   A group of small nerve cell bodies about the size of a cherry, located along the base of the brain beneath the thalamus. In addition to exerting control over the sympathetic nervous system, the hypothalamus also controls several vital body functions, including temperature, sleep cycle, sexual behavior, and respiratory activity. The hypothalamus also coordinates the function of the endocrine system.

Hypothyroidism   Underactivity of the thyroid gland, resulting in underproduction of thyroid hormones.

Iatrogenic   Literally meaning "physician produced," this term refers to any condition, disease, or other adverse occurrence that results from medical treatment.

Ictal   The period of the actual seizure itself.

Infantile seizures   Seizures seen in early childhood (infants through age 4) consisting of 1 to 4 seconds of tonic-like movements with arms flung forward or outward.

Insulin   A hormone produced by the pancreas in response to the level of glucose in the blood. Insulin promotes the absorption of glucose into the cells, where it is converted into energy.

inter-   A prefix meaning *between.*

Interictal   The weeks or months between seizures.

ipsi-   Prefix meaning *the same.*

Ipsilateral   On the same side.

Islet of Langerhans   The cells in the pancreas that produce insulin.

-itis   Suffix meaning *inflammation of.*

Jacksonian march   A specific type of seizure that generally begins with either a tonic spasm or a clonic rhythmic twitching of the fingers of one hand, or face on one side, and so on. The seizure then spreads in a progressive march—for example, from face to neck to hand and forearm to trunk to leg, all on one side. These seizures may also be sensory in nature.

-kinesia   Suffix meaning *having to do with movement.*

-lexia   Suffix meaning *having to do with reading.*

Limbic system   A ring-shaped area in the center of the brain, consisting of connected clusters of nerve cells, that plays a role in the autonomic nervous system, the emotions, and the sense of smell. The hippocampus, cingulate and hippocampal gyri, and amygdala are all part of the limbic system.

macro-   Prefix meaning *large.*

Macroscopia   An elementary visual illusion in which objects appear larger than they actually are.

Magnetic resonance imaging (MRI)   A diagnostic method that provides high-quality cross-sectional images of organs and structures in the body without using X rays or radiation. The patient is exposed to short bursts of powerful magnetic fields and radio waves, which stimulate the hydrogen atoms in the patient's tissues to emit signals. These signals are detected and analyzed by computer to create an image of a "slice" of a person's body.

Microscopia   An elementary visual illusion in which objects appear smaller than they actually are.

Mitral valve prolapse   A common, slight deformity of the mitral valve in the left side of the heart, most commonly seen among young to middle-aged women. There is a characteristic heart murmur that can usually be heard through a stethoscope during routine examination.

Multiple endocrine neoplasia syndromes   The co-occurrence of more than one endocrine disorder characterized by overproduction of a hormone.

Multiple sclerosis   A progressive disease of the central nervous system in which patches of myelin in the brain and spinal cord are destroyed, resulting in symptoms ranging from numbness and tingling to paralysis and incontinence.

Myelin   The fatty material that forms a protective sheath around some types of nerve fibers and acts as an electrical insulator, increasing the efficiency of nerve impulse conduction.

Myoclonic seizures   Seizures characterized by rapid, uncontrollable jerks or spasms of muscles.

Myxedema madness   A severe form of psychosis resulting from untreated hypothyroidism.

Necrotic   Characterized by dead tissue cells.

Neurotransmitter   A chemical that transmits the electrical impulse from one neuron to another. Many of these are similar or identical to chemicals used by the body as hormones.

Norepinephrine   A hormone secreted by the adrenal glands (and by nerve endings in the sympathetic nervous system). The primary function of this hormone is to help maintain a constant blood pressure.

Olfactory   Having to do with the sense of smell.

Olfactory hallucination   The fleeting perception of a strange smell that is a primictal event.

Paliacousia   A neurological symptom in which the patient seizes on a word or words and then hears them over and over again in a hallucinatory manner.

Paralinguistics The unspoken communication in language. This includes things such as tone of voice and inflections.

Parathyroid glands Two pairs of pea-sized glands located adjacent to the two lobes of the thyroid gland. These glands produce parathyroid hormone, which helps regulate the amount of calcium in the blood.

Paroxysmal Caused by a seizure; sudden and episodic.

Partial seizures Seizures that occur in only a small, focused portion of the brain.

Pathology The nature of diseases, particularly the structural and functional changes caused by the disease.

-pathy A suffix denoting a disease or disorder.

Peripheral neuropathy Damage, disease, or inflammation of the peripheral nerves, those nerves that connect the central nervous system to the sense organs, muscles, internal organs, and glands.

Petit mal seizure A seizure common in children and adolescents, characterized by a momentary loss of awareness, such that an observer might believe the child is daydreaming.

Pheochromocytoma A tumor on the adrenal medulla resulting in increased production of epinephrine and norepinephrine.

Pituitary gland A pea-sized structure hanging from the base of the brain just below the optic nerves, this "master gland" regulates and controls the activities of other endocrine glands and many body processes.

Polyglandular insufficiency syndrome The co-occurrence of more than one endocrine disorder characterized by underproduction of a hormone.

Poriomania A condition occurring during a prolonged ictal period during which the patient wanders off and engages in ordinary, stereotyped activities without consciousness. The patient later "wakes up" having lost time.

Posterior Relating to the back of the body. In humans, this is synonymous with *dorsal.*

Posterolateral sclerosis A neurological disorder involving progressive degeneration of the lateral and posterior columns of the spinal cord and peripheral nerves.

Postictal The minutes and hours just after a seizure.

Postural seizure This type of elementary focal seizure involves a tonic posturing of a part of the body.

Primictal The minutes before the actual seizure.

Prodromal Warning symptoms indicating the onset of an illness. In the case of seizure disorders, the prodromal stage can begin hours or days before the seizure.

Prolapse Displacement of all or a portion of an organ or tissue from its normal position.

Proprioceptive Information the body uses to determine its position relative to the outside world and the state of contraction of its muscles.

Psychomotor epilepsy Another term for complex partial seizures or temporal lobe epilepsy.

Putamen Brain structure that is part of the basil ganglia, the portion of the extrapyramidal nervous system that is responsible for coordination, especially the control of automatic associated movements.

Red nucleus One of three brain structures located in the upper midbrain that works in close association with the basil ganglia and is considered part of the extrapyramidal nervous system.

Seizure   A sudden episode of abnormal electrical activity in the brain. The location and magnitude of the abnormal electrical discharge determines the symptoms exhibited by the patient. Recurrent seizures are called epilepsy.

Septal nuclei   A subcortical brain structure that is part of the limbic system.

somata-   A prefix meaning *related to the body*.

Somatosensory seizure   This type of elementary focal seizure originates in the sensory strip of the parietal lobe and consists of tingling sensations and pins-and-needles sensations in a part of the body contralateral to the discharging focus.

stereo-   Prefix meaning *touch*.

Stereognosis   The ability to recognize objects by touch alone.

Substantia nigra   A structure located in the brain stem. Lesions in this structure produce muscular rigidity, a resting tremor, a slow, shuffling gait, and a masklike facial appearance. Parkinson's disease affects this structure.

Systemic lupus erythematosus   A chronic autoimmune disorder that causes inflammation of connective tissue. It affects many systems of the body, including the joints and kidneys.

Systole   The period of muscular contraction in the heart that alternates with the resting period (diastole). The contractions pump blood out of the heart into the arteries.

Tachycardia   Rapid heart rate, usually defined as greater than 100 beats per minute in an adult.

Tardive dyskinesia   One of the drug-induced extrapyramidal syndromes, this irreversible collection of symptoms is the result of the use of antipsychotic medication and occurs in 10% to 20% of patients maintained on phenothiazines for an extended period of time.

-taxia   Suffix meaning *coordination*.

Temporal lobe epilepsy   A form of epilepsy in which the abnormal electrical discharges are localized in the temporal region of the brain. Because the temporal lobes are concerned with functions such as smell, taste, hearing, visual associations, and some elements of memory, the abnormal discharges may cause disruptions in any of these areas.

Tetany   Spasms and twitching of the muscles most commonly in the hands, feet, face, and larynx. The most common cause of tetany is hypocalcemia (often due to a diet lacking in Vitamin D), which can also result from hypoparathyroidism.

Thalamus   A pair of walnut-sized structures located deep within the brain that serves as an important relay center for sensory information flowing into the brain. The thalamus appears to act as a filter, selecting only information of particular importance from the mass of sensory signals entering the brain.

Thyroid panel   Blood tests used to evaluate the functioning of the thyroid gland. The levels of thyroxine (T_4) and triiodothyronine (T_3) are obtained.

Tonic phase   The initial portion of a grand mal seizure during which there is an abrupt loss of consciousness and a stiffening of the body.

Tonic seizure   A seizure consisting of brief stiffening and extension of the limbs that is associated with a fast EEG pattern. These are seen most often in children with Lennox-Gastaut syndrome.

Toxins   Poisons.

Transverse temporal gyrus   Also called Heschl's area. Auditory impulses to the brain are represented here.

Vertiginous sensory seizure This type of seizure arises from the superior temporal gyrus and produces a whirling-spinning sensation that can be very nauseating.

Vestibular Concerned with balance.

Viscosity One of the characteristics of the interictal stage in patients with temporal lobe epilepsy (complex partial seizures) during which the patient adheres to each thought, feeling, or activity and is overinclusive and gives excessive detail in his or her speech.

Visual sensory seizure This type of seizure occurs with discharge in the occipital lobe and is characterized by unformed visual hallucinations, such as flashing lights or colors, or by a dimming of vision in the contralateral visual field.

Volitional movement Voluntary, purposeful movement.

Wilson's disease An inherited disorder involving the excessive absorption of copper along with decreased excretion of copper by the liver. Copper then builds up in the liver and brain, creating psychiatric, neurological, and physical symptoms.

Bibliography

Chapter 1

Brown, G. M. (1975). Psychiatric and neurologic aspects of endocrine disease. *Hospital Practice, 10,* 71-79.

Hershman, J. M. (1980). *Management of endocrine disorders.* Philadelphia: Lea Febiger.

Morley, J. E. (1983). The aging endocrine system. *Postgraduate Medicine, 73,* 107-120.

Morley, J. E., & Krahn, D. D. (1987). Endocrinology for the psychiatrist. In C. B. Nemeroff & P. T. Loosen (Eds.), *Handbook of clinical psychoneuroendocrinology* (pp. 3-37). New York: Guilford.

Popkin, M. K., & MacKenzie, T. B. (1980). Psychiatric presentations of endocrine dysfunction. In R. C. W. Hall (Ed.), *Psychiatric presentations of medical illnesses* (pp. 139-156). New York: Spectrum.

Sacher, E. J. (1976). *Hormones, behavior and psychopathology.* New York: Raven.

Scanlon, M. F. (1983). Neuroendocrinology. *Clinics in Endocrinology and Metabolism, 12,* 467-858.

Smith, C. K., Barish, J., Correa, J., & Williams, R. H. (1972). Psychiatric disturbance in endocrinologic disease. *Psychosomatic Medicine, 34,* 69-86.

Whybrow, P. C., & Hurwitz, T. (1976). Psychological disturbances associated with endocrine disease and hormone therapy. In E. J. Sacker (Ed.), *Hormones, behavior and psychopathology* (pp. 125-144). New York: Raven.

Wurtman, R. J., & Fernstrom, J. D. (1976). Neuroendocrine effects of psychotropic drugs. In E. J. Sacher (Ed.), *Hormones, behavior and psychopathology* (pp. 145-152). New York: Raven.

Chapter 2

Bagchi, N., Brown, T., & Mack, R. (1982). Effect of chronic lithium treatment on hypothalamic-pituitary regulation of thyroid function. *Hormone and Metabolic Research, 14,* 92-93.

Barnes, V., Greenberg, A., et al. (1972). The effect of chlordiazepoxide on thyroid function and thyrotoxicosis. *Johns Hopkins Medical Journal, 131,* 298-300.

Bauer, M. S., Whybrow, P. C., & Winokur, A. (1990). Rapid cycling bipolar affective disorder 1. Association with grade 1 hypothyroidism. *Archives of General Psychiatry, 47*(5), 427-432.

Beyer, J., Burke, M., Meglin, D., Fuller, A., Krishnan, K. R., & Nemeroff, C. B. (1993). Organic anxiety disorder: Iatrogenic hyperthyroidism. *Psychosomatics, 34*(2), 181-184.

Blum, M. (1972). Myxedema coma. *American Journal of the Medical Sciences, 264,* 432-443.

Bommer, M., & Naber, D. (1992). Subclinical hypothyroidism in recurrent mania. *Biological psychiatry, 31*(7), 729-734.

Cho, J., Bone, S., et al. (1979). The effect of lithium on thyroid function in patients with primary affective disorder. *American Journal of Psychiatry, 136,* 115-116.

Clarnette, R. M., & Patterson, C. J. (1994). Hypothyroidism: Does treatment cure dementia? *Journal of Geriatric Psychiatry and Neurology, 7*(1), 23-27.

Cohen, K., & Swigar, M. (1979). Thyroid function screening in psychiatric patients. *JAMA, 242,* 254-257.

Cooper, D., Halpern, R., et al. (1984). Thyroxine therapy in subclinical hypothyroidism. *Annals of Internal Medicine, 101,* 18-24.

Crocker, A., & Overstreet, D. (1984). Modification of the behavioral effects of haloperidol and of dopamine receptor regulation by altered thyroid status. *Psychopharmacology, 82,* 102-106.

Drinka, P. J., & Voeks, S. K. (1987). Psychological depressive symptoms in grade II hypothyroidism in a nursing home. *Psychiatry Research, 21,* 199-204.

Extein, I., Pottash, A., & Gold, M. (1982). Does subclinical hypothyroidism predispose to tricyclic-induced rapid mood cycles? *Journal of Clinical Psychiatry, 43,* 290-291.

Fava, M., Labbate, L. A., Abraham, M. E., & Rosenbaum, J. F. (1995). Hypothyroidism and hyperthyroidism in major depression revisited. *Journal of Clinical Psychiatry, 56*(5), 186-192.

Fonseca, V., Wakeling, A., & Havard, C. W. H. (1990). Hyperthyroidism and eating disorders. *British Medical Journal, 301*(6747), 322-323.

Haggerty, J. J., Jr., & Prange, A. J., Jr. (1995). Borderline hypothyroidism and depression. *Annual Review of Medicine, 46,* 37-46.

Haggerty, J. J., Jr., Stern, R. A., Mason, G. A., Beckwith, J., Morey, C. E., & Prange, A. J., Jr. (1993). Subclinical hypothyroidism: A modifiable risk factor for depression? *American Journal of Psychiatry, 150*(3), 508-510.

Josephson, A., & MacKenzie, T. (1980). Thyroid-induced mania in hypothyroid patients. *British Journal of Psychiatry, 137,* 222-228.

Morley, J. E., Shafer, R. B., et al. (1980). Amphetamine-induced hyperthyroidism. *Annals of Internal Medicine, 93,* 707-709.

Peake, P. (1981). Recurrent apathetic hypothyroidism. *Archives of Internal Medicine, 141,* 258-262.

Perrild, H., Madson, S., & Hansen, J. (1978). Irreversible myxedema after lithium carbonate. *British Medical Journal, 1,* 1108-1109.

Reisberg, B., & Gershon, S. (1979). Side effects associated with lithium therapy. *Archives of General Psychiatry, 36,* 879-887.

Schader, R., & DiMascio, A. (1970). *Psychotropic drug side effects.* Baltimore: Williams & Wilkins.

Shen, F., & Sherrard, D. J. (1982). Lithium-induced hyperparathyroidism. *Annals of Internal Medicine, 96,* 63-65.

Steinberg, P. I. (1994). A case of paranoid disorder associated with hypothyroidism. *Canadian Journal of Psychiatry, 39,* 153-156.

Swanson, J., Kelly, J., & McConahey, W. (1981). Neurologic aspects of thyroid dysfunction. *Mayo Clinic Proceedings, 56,* 504-512.

Taylor, J. (1975). Depression in thyrotoxicosis. *American Journal of Psychiatry, 132,* 552-554.

Trzepacz, P. T., McCue, M., Klein, I., Levey, G. S., & Greenhouse, J. (1988). A psychiatric and neuropsychological study of patients with untreated Graves' disease. *General Hospital Psychiatry, 10,* 49-55.

Wallace, J., MacCrimmon, D., & Goldberg, W. (1980). Acute hyperthyroidism: Cognitive and emotional correlates. *Journal of Abnormal Psychology, 89,* 519-527.

Weiner, M. (1979). Haloperidol, hyperthyroidism and sudden death. *American Journal of Psychiatry, 136,* 717-718.

Witschy, J., & Redmond, F. (1981). Extrapyramidal reaction to fluphenazine potentiated by thyrotoxicosis. *American Journal of Psychiatry, 138,* 246-249.

Chapter 3

Adrenal Disorders: Addison's Disease

Brown, G. M. (1974). Psychiatric and neurologic aspects of endocrine disease. *Hospital Practice, 10,* 71-79.

DeMilio, L., Dakis, C. A., et al. (1984). Addison's disease initially diagnosed as bereavement and conversion disorder. *American Journal of Psychiatry, 141,* 1647-1648.

Hall, R. C. W., Popkin, M. K., et al. (1979). Presentation of the steroid psychoses. *Journal of Nervous and Mental Disease, 167,* 229-236.

Lewis, D. A., & Smith, R. E. (1983). Steroid-induced psychiatric syndromes. *Journal of Affective Disorders, 5,* 319-332.

Money, J., & Jobaris, R. (1977). Juvenile Addison's disease. *Psychoneuroendocrinology, 2,* 147-157.

Ur, E., Turner, T. H., Goodwin, T. J., Grossman, A., & Besser, G. M. (1992). Mania in association with hydrocortisone replacement for Addison's disease. *Postgraduate Medical Journal, 68*(795), 41-43.

Adrenal Disorders: Cushing's Syndrome

Aron, D. C., Tyrrell, J. B., et al. (1981). Cushing's syndrome: Problems in diagnosis. *Medicine, 60,* 25-35.

Becker, L., Gold, P., & Chrousos, G. (1983). Analogies between Cushing's disease and depression. *General Hospital Psychiatry, 5,* 89-91.

Cohen, S. I. (1980). Cushing's syndrome: A psychiatric study of 29 patients. *British Journal of Psychiatry, 136,* 120-124.

Gold, E. M. (1979). The Cushing syndromes. *Annals of Internal Medicine, 90,* 829-844.

Heinz, E. R., Martinez, J., & Haenggeli, A. (1977). Reversibility of cerebral atrophy in anorexia nervosa and Cushing's syndrome. *Journal of Computer Assisted Tomography, 1,* 415-418.

Jeffcoate, W., Silverstone, J., et al. (1979). Psychiatric manifestations of Cushing's syndrome. *Quarterly Journal of Medicine, 43,* 465-472.

Kelly, W. F., Checkley, S. A., & Bender, D. A. (1980). Cushing's syndrome, tryptophan and depression. *British Journal of Psychiatry, 136,* 125-132.

Krystal, A., Krishnan, K. R., Raitiere, M., Poland, R., Ritchie, J. C., et al. (1990). Differential diagnosis and psychopathology of Cushing's syndrome and primary affective disorder. *Journal of Neuropsychiatry and Clinical Neuroscience, 2,* 34-43.

Loosen, P. T., Chambliss, B., DeBold, C. R., Shelton, R., & Orth, D. N. (1992). Psychiatric phenomenology in Cushing's disease. *Pharmacopsychiatry, 25,* 192-198.

Reed, K., Watkins, M., & Dobson, H. (1983). Mania in Cushing's syndrome. *Journal of Clinical Psychiatry, 44,* 460-462.

Sonino, N., Fava, G. A., Belluardo, P., Girelli, M. E., & Boscaro, M. (1993). Course of depression in Cushing's syndrome: Response to treatment and comparison with Graves' disease. *Hormone Research, 39*(5/6), 202-206.

Storkman, M. N., Schteingart, D. E., & Schork, M. A. (1981). Depressed mood and other psychiatric manifestations of Cushing's syndrome. *Psychosomatic Medicine, 43,* 3-18.

Pituitary Disorders

Gutowski, N. J., & Heron, J. R. (1993). Recurrent confusion and hypopituitarism. *Postgraduate Medical Journal, 69*(811), 392-394.

Lynch, S., Merson, S., Beshyah, S. A., Skinner, E., Sharp, P., Priest, R. G., & Johnston, D. G. (1994). Psychiatric morbidity in adults with hypopituitarism. *Journal of the Royal Society of Medicine, 87*(8), 445-447.

Parathyroid Disorders

Alarcon, R. D., & Franceschini, J. A. (1984). Hyperparathyroidism and paranoid psychosis. *British Journal of Psychiatry, 145,* 477-486.

Borer, M. S., & Bhanot, U. K. (1985). Hyperparathyroidism: Neuropsychiatric manifestations. *Psychosomatics, 26,* 597-601.

Cope, D. (1960). Hyperparathyroidism: Diagnosis and management. *American Journal of Surgery, 99,* 394-403.

Denko, J. D., & Koebling, R. (1962). The psychiatric aspects of hypoparathyroidism. *Acta Psychiatrica Scandinavica, 164*(Suppl.), 5-38.

Flanagan, T. A., Goodwin, D. W., et al. (1970). Psychiatric illness in a large family with familial hyperparathyroidism. *British Journal of Psychiatry, 117,* 693-698.

Franks, R. D., Dubovsky, S. L., et al. (1982). Long-term lithium carbonate therapy causes hyperparathyroidism. *Archives of General Psychiatry, 39,* 1074-1077.

Gold, M., Pottash, A., & Extein, I. (1981). Hypoparathyroidism and depression. *JAMA, 245,* 1919-1921.

Heath, H., Hodgson, S. F., & Kennedy, M. A. (1980). Primary hyperparathyroidism: Incidence, morbidity and potential economic impact in a community. *New England Journal of Medicine, 302,* 189-193.

Kingsbury, S. J., & Salzman, C. (1993). Psychopharmacology: Lithium's role in hyperparathyroidism and hypercalcemia. *Hospital and Community Psychiatry, 44*(11), 1047-1048.

Mallette, L. E. (1992). Hypoparathyroidism with menses-associated hypocalcemia. *American Journal of the Medical Sciences, 304*(1), 32-37.

Peterson, P. (1968). Psychiatric disorders in primary hyperparathyroidism. *Journal of Clinical Endocrinology, 28,* 1491-1495.

Tonner, D. R., & Schlechter, J. A. (1993). Neurologic complications of thyroid and parathyroid disease. *Medical Clinics of North America, 77,* 251-263.

Chapter 5

Berrios, G. E., Campbell, C., & Politynska, B. E. (1995). Autonomic failure, depression and anxiety in Parkinson's disease. *British Journal of Psychiatry, 166,* 789-792.

Brodal, A. (1981). *Neurological anatomy in relation to clinical medicine.* London: Oxford University Press.

Carpenter, M. B., & Sutin, J. (1983). *Human neuroanatomy.* Baltimore: Williams & Wilkins.

DeJong, R. N., & Sugar, O. (1971). *The yearbook of neurology and neurosurgery.* Chicago: Yearbook Medical Publishers.

Hantz, P., Caradoc-Davies, G., Caradoc-Davies, T., Weatherall, M., & Dixon, G. (1994). Depression in Parkinson's disease. *American Journal of Psychiatry, 151,* 1010-1014.

Haymaker, W. (1985). *Bing's local diagnosis in neurological disease.* St. Louis, MO: C. V. Mosby.

Miller, C. H., Simioni, I., Oberbauer, H., Schwitzer, J., Batnas, C., Kulhanek, F., Boissel, K. E., Meise, U., Hinterhuber, H., & Fleischhacker, W. (1995). Tardive dyskinesia prevalence rates during a ten-year follow-up. *Journal of Nervous and Mental Disease, 183*(6), 404-407.

Starkstein, S. E., Robinson, R. G., & Leiguarda, R. (1993). Anxiety and depression in Parkinson's disease. *Behavioral Neurology, 6,* 151-154.

Sweet, R. A., Mulsant, B. H., Gupta, B., Rifai, A. H., Pasternak, R. E., McEachran, A., & Zubenko, G. S. (1995). Duration of neuroleptic treatment and prevalence of tardive dyskinesia in late life. *Archives of General Psychiatry, 52*(6), 478-486.

Chapter 6

DeJong, R. N., & Sugar, O. (1971). *The yearbook of neurology and neurosurgery.* Chicago: Yearbook Medical Publishers.

Erkwoh, R. (1990). Psychopathology of vestibular aurae. *Psychopathology, 23,* 129-135.

Gazzaniga, M. (1979). *Handbook of behavioral neurobiology and neuropsychology.* New York: Plenum.

Livingston, S. (1971). *Comprehensive management of epilepsy in infancy, childhood, and adolescence.* Springfield, IL: Charles C Thomas.

Penfield, W., & Jasper, H. (1954). *Epilepsy and the functional anatomy of the human brain.* Boston: Little, Brown.

Chapter 7

The bibliography for this chapter is arranged by symptoms of temporal lobe epilepsy rather than by the stages of a complex partial seizure denoted by chapter headings.

General Information

Bear, D. (1979a). Temporal lobe epilepsy: A syndrome of sensory-limbic hyperconnection. *Cortex, 15,* 357-384.

Bear, D. (1979b). The temporal lobes: An approach to the study of organic behavioral changes. In M. Gazzaniga (Ed.), *Handbook of behavioral neurobiology, and neuropsychology.* New York: Plenum.

Bear, D., & Fedio, P. (1977). Quantitative analysis of interictal behavior in temporal lobe epilepsy. *Archives of Neurology, 34,* 454-467.

Benson, D. F., & Blumer D. (Eds.). (1975). *Psychiatric aspects of neurologic disease.* New York: Grune & Stratton.

Blumer, D. (1971). Neuropsychiatric aspects of psychomotor and other forms of epilepsy. In S. Livingston (Ed.), *Comprehensive management of epilepsy in infancy, childhood, and adolescence.* Springfield, IL: Charles C Thomas.

Cascino, G. D. (1992). Complex partial seizures: Clinical features and differential diagnosis. *Psychiatric Clinics of North America, 15*(2), 101-118.

Fiordelli, E., Beghi, E., Bogliun, G., & Crespi, V. (1993). Epilepsy and psychiatric disturbance. *British Journal of Psychiatry, 163,* 446-450.

McNeil, T. F., Wiegerink, R., & Dozier, J. E. (1970). Pregnancy and birth complications in the births of seriously, moderately, and mildly behaviorally disturbed children. *Journal of Nervous and Mental Disease, 151*(1), 24-30.

Ounsted, C. et al. (1966). *Biological factors in temporal lobe epilepsy*. London: Heinemann.

Ounsted, C., & Lindsay, J. (1982). The long-term outcome of temporal lobe epilepsy in childhood. In E. H. Reynolds & M. R. Trimble (Eds.), *Psychiatry and epilepsy* (pp. 185-215). London: Churchill Livingstone.

Penfield W. et al. (1954). *Epilepsy and the functional anatomy of the human brain*. Boston: Little Brown.

Sexual Behavior and Disorders

Blumer, D., & Walker, A. E. (1967). Sexual behavior in temporal lobe epilepsy. *Archives of Neurology, 16*, 37-43.

Blumer, D. (1970). Hypersexual episodes in temporal lobe epilepsy. *American Journal of Psychiatry, 126*, 1099-1106.

Himmelhock, J. A. (1989). Hypersexuality in temporal lobe epilepsy. *Medical Aspects of Human Sexuality, 23*(11), 56-64.

Hooshmand, H. et al. (1969). Temporal lobe seizures and exhibitionism. *Neurology, 19*, 1119-1124.

Taylor, D. C. (1969). Sexual behavior and temporal lobe epilepsy. *Archives of Neurology, 21*, 510-516.

Temporal Lobe Personality

Blumer, D. (1975). Temporal lobe epilepsy and its psychiatric significance. In D. F. Benson & D. Blumer (Eds.), *Psychiatric aspects of neurologic disease*. New York: Grune & Stratton.

Blumer, D. (1977, June). Treatment of patients with seizure disorder referred because of psychiatric complications. *McLean Hospital Journal*, pp. 53-73.

Dewhurst, K. et al. (1970). Sudden religious conversions in temporal lobe epilepsy. *British Journal of Psychiatry, 117*, 497-507.

Waxman, S. G., & Geschwind, N. (1974). Hypergraphia in temporal lobe epilepsy. *Neurology, 24*, 629-636.

Depression, Anxiety, and Other Symptoms

Altshuler, L. L., Devinsky, O., Post, R. M., & Theodore, W. (1990). Depression, anxiety and temporal lobe epilepsy. *Archives of Neurology, 47*(3), 284-288.

Blumer, D. (1977, June). Treatment of patients with seizure disorder referred because of psychiatric complications. *McLean Hospital Journal*, pp. 53-73.

Devinsky, O., & Vasquez, B. (1993). Behavioral changes associated with epilepsy. *Neurologic Clinics, 11*(1), 127-149.

Erkwoh, R. (1990). Psychopathology of vestibular aurae. *Psychopathology, 23*(3), 129-135.

Hambert, G., & Willen, R. (1978). Emotional disturbance and temporal lobe injury. *Comprehensive Psychiatry, 19*(5), 441-447.

Indaco, A., Carrieri, P. B., Nappi, C., Gentile, S., & Striano, S. (1992). Interictal depression in epilepsy. *Epilepsy Research, 12*(1), 45-50.

Mayeux, R. et al. (1979). Poriomania. *Neurology, 29*, 1616-1619.

Mendez, M. F., & Doss, R. C. (1992). Ictal and psychiatric aspects of suicide in epileptic patients. *International Journal of Psychiatry and Medicine, 22*, 231-237.

Mendez, M. F., Doss, R. C., Taylor, J. L., & Salguero, P. (1993). Depression and epilepsy. *Journal of Nervous and Mental Disease, 181*(7), 444-447.

Mendez, M. F., Taylor, J. L., Doss, R. C., & Salguero, P. (1994). Depression in secondary epilepsy: Relation to lesion laterality. *Journal of Neurology, Neurosurgery and Psychiatry, 57*(2), 232-233.

Seidenberg, M., Herman, B., & Wyler, A. R. (1995). Depression in temporal lobe epilepsy. *Neuropsychiatry, Neuropsychology and Behavior, 8*(2), 81-87.

Septien, L., Giroud, M., Didi-Roy, R., Pelletier, J. L., Marin, A., & Dumas, R. (1993). Depression and partial epilepsy. *Neurological Research, 15*(2), 136-138.

Silberman, E. K., Sussman, N., Skillings, G., & Callanan, M. (1994). Aura phenomena and psychopathology. *Epilepsia, 35,* 778-784.

Spitz, M. C. (1991). Panic disorder in seizure patients: A diagnostic pitfall. *Epilepsia, 32,* 33-38.

The Schizophrenia-Like Interictal Psychosis

Bruton, C. J., Stevens, J. R., & Frith, C. D. (1994). Epilepsy, psychosis, and schizophrenia: Clinical and neuropathologic correlations. *Neurology, 44*(1), 34-42.

Flor-Henry, P. (1969). Psychosis and temporal lobe epilepsy: A controlled investigation. *Epilepsia, 10,* 363-395.

Hecaen, H., & Albert, M. L. (1978a). Auditory illusions and hallucinations. In H. Hecaen & M. L. Albert (Eds.), *Human neuropsychology* (pp. 257-276). New York: John Wiley.

Hecaen, H., & Albert, M. L. (1978b). Visual illusions and hallucinations. In H. Hecaen & M. L. Albert (Eds.), *Human neuropsychology* (pp. 144-165). New York: John Wiley.

Kristensen, O., & Sindrup, E. H. (1978). Psychomotor epilepsy and psychosis. *Acta Neuroligica Scandinavica, 57,* 361-370.

Mendez, M. F., Grau, R., Doss, R. C., & Taylor, J. L. (1993). Schizophrenia in epilepsy: Seizure and psychosis variables. *Neurology, 43*(6), 1073-1077.

Perez, M. M., & Trimble, M. R. (1980). Epileptic psychosis: Diagnostic comparison with process schizophrenia. *British Journal of Psychiatry, 137,* 245-249.

Slater, E., & Beard, A. W. (1963). The schizophrenia-like psychosis of epilepsy. *British Journal of Psychiatry, 109,* 95-150.

Taylor, J. (1931). *Selected writings of Hughlings Jackson* (Vols. 1 & 2). London: Hodder & Stoughton.

Toone, B. (1982). Psychoses of epilepsy. In E. H. Reynolds & M. R. Trimble (Eds.), *Psychiatry and epilepsy.* London: Churchill Livingstone.

Antisocial, Violent, and Delinquent Behaviors

Andrulonis, P. A. (1980). Preliminary data on ethosuximide and the episodic dyscontrol syndrome. *American Journal of Psychiatry, 137,* 1455-1456.

Bach-Y-Rita, G. et al. (1971). Episodic dyscontrol: A study of 130 violent patients. *American Journal of Psychiatry, 127,* 1473-1478.

Berman, A. (1972). Neurological dysfunction in juvenile delinquency: Implications for early intervention. *Child Care Quarterly, 1*(4), 164-271.

Berman, A., & Siegal, A. (1976). A neuropsychological approach to the etiology, prevention, and treatment of juvenile delinquency. In A. Davids (Ed), *Child personality and psychopathology: Current topics* (Vol 3). New York: John Wiley.

Blumer, D. (1976). Epilepsy and violence. In D. J. Madder & J. Lion (Eds.), *Rage, hate, assault and other forms of violence.* New York: Spectrum.

Cantwell, D. P. (1978). Hyperactivity and antisocial behavior. *Journal of the American Academy of Child Psychiatry, 17,* 252-262.

Elliot, F. A. (1978). Neurological aspects of antisocial behavior. In W. Reid (Ed.), *The psychopath: A comprehensive study of antisocial disorder and behaviors.* New York: Brunner-Mazel.

Fedio, P., & Mirsky, A. F. (1969). Selective intellectual deficits in children with temporal lobe or centrencephalic epilepsy. *Neuropsychologia, 7*(4), 287-300.

Geschwind, N. (1975). The clinical setting of aggression in temporal lobe epilepsy. In Fields & Sweet (Eds), *The neurobiology of violence.* St. Louis, MO: Warren H. Green.

Girgis, M., & Kiloh, L. G. (1980). *Limbic epilepsy and dyscontrol syndrome.* Amsterdam: Elsevier.

Greenberg, I. M. (1970). Clinical correlates of 14 and 6 cycles per second positive EEG spiking and family pathology. *Journal of Abnormal Psychology, 76*(3), 403-412.

Gross, M. D., & Wilson, W. C. (1964). Behavior disorders of children with cerebral dysrhythmia. *Archives of General Psychiatry, 11,* 610-619.

Klinfman, D. et al. (1975). Temporal lobe epilepsy and aggression. *Journal of Nervous and Mental Disease, 160,* 324-341.

Krynicki, V. E. (1978). Cerebral dysfunction in repetitively assaultive adolescents. *Journal of Nervous and Mental Disease, 166,* 59-67.

Lewis, D. O. (1976). Delinquency, psychomotor epilepsy symptoms, and paranoid ideation: A triad. *American Journal of Psychiatry, 133,* 1395-1398.

Maletzky, B. M. (1973). The episodic dyscontrol syndrome. *Diseases of the Nervous System, 36,* 178-185.

Mendez, M. F., Doss, R. C., & Taylor, J. L. (1993). Interictal violence in epilepsy: Relationship to behavior and seizure variables. *Journal of Nervous and Mental Disease, 181*(9), 566-569.

Pincus, J. H. (1980). Can violence be a manifestation of epilepsy? *Neurology, 30,* 304-307.

Quitkin, F. et al. (1976). Neurologic soft signs in schizophrenia and character disorders. *Archives of General Psychiatry, 33,* 845-847.

Reitan, R. M., & Heineman, C. E. (1968). Interactions of neurological deficits and emotional disturbances in children with learning disorders: Methods for differential assessment. In *Learning disorders* (Vol. 3). Seattle, WA: Special Child Publications.

Rodin, E. A. (1973). Psychomotor epilepsy and aggressive behavior. *Archives of General Psychiatry, 28,* 210-215.

Schwade, E. D., & Geiger, S. G. (1953). Matricide with EEG evidence of thalamic or hypothalamic disorder. *Diseases of the Nervous System, 14,* 18-20.

Schwade, E. D., & Geiger, S. G. (1960). Severe behavior disorders with abnormal EEGs. *Diseases of the Nervous System, 21,* 616-620.

Serafetinides, E. A. (1965). Aggressiveness in temporal lobe epileptics and its relation to cerebral dysfunction and environmental factors. *Epilepsia, 6,* 33-42.

Small, J. G. (1964). 14 and 6 per second positive spikes. *Archives of General Psychiatry, 11,* 645-650.

Stevens, J. R. et al. (1981). Temporal lobe epilepsy, psychopathology, and violence: The state of the evidence. *Neurology, 31,* 1127-1132.

Walter, R. D. (1960). Controlled study of 14 and 6 per second EEG pattern. *Archives of General Psychiatry, 2,* 559-566.

Weiner, J. H. et al. (1966). An EEG study of delinquents and non-delinquents. *Archives of General Psychiatry, 15,* 144-150.

Winfield, D. L., & Ozturk, O. (1959). EEG findings in matricide: A case report. *Diseases of the Nervous System, 20,* 176-178.

Woods, S. M. (1964). Adolescent violence and homicide: Ego disruption and the 6-14 dysrthymia. *Archives of General Psychiatry, 5,* 528-534.

Effects of Psychiatric Drugs

Mendez, M. F., Cummings, J. L., & Benson, D. F. (1986). Psychotropic drugs and epilepsy. *Stress Medicine, 2,* 325-332.

Thompson, P. J., & Trimble, M. R. (1982). Anticonvulsant drugs and cognitive functions. *Epilepsia, 23,* 531-544.

Toone, B. K., & Fenton, G. W. (1977). Epileptic seizures induced by psychotropic drugs. *Psychological Medicine, 7,* 265-270.

Trimble, M. R. (1978). Non-MAOI antidepressants and epilepsy. A review. *Epilepsia, 19,* 241-250.

Chapter 8

Multiple Sclerosis

Arias Bal, M. A., Vazquez-Barquero, J. L., Peqa, C., Miro, J., & Berciano, J. A. (1991). Psychiatric aspects of multiple sclerosis. *Acta Psychiatrica Scandinavica, 83*(4), 292-296.

Bezkor, M. F., & Canedo, A. (1987). Physiological and psychological factors influencing sexual dysfunction in multiple sclerosis: Part I. *Sexuality and Disability, 8*(3), 143-146.

Boyle, E. A., Clark, C. M., Klonoff, H., Paty, D. W., & Oger, J. (1991). Empirical support for psychological profiles observed in multiple sclerosis. *Archives of Neurology, 48*(11), 1150-1154.

Burnfield, A. et al. (1978). Common psychological problems in multiple sclerosis. *British Medical Journal,* 1193-1194.

Freyne, A., & Shelley, R. K. (1994). Obsessive compulsive disorder and multiple sclerosis. *Irish Journal of Psychological Medicine, 11*(1), 26.

Hotopf, M. H., Pollock, S., & Lishman, W. A. (1994). An unusual presentation of multiple sclerosis. *Psychological Medicine, 24*(2), 525-528.

Ivnik, R. J. (1978). Neuropsychological test performance as a function of duration of multiple sclerosis-related symptomatology. *Journal of Clinical Psychology, 39,* 311-331.

Mahler, M. E. (1992). Behavioral manifestations associated with multiple sclerosis. *Psychiatric Clinics of North America, 15*(2), 427-438.

Marsh, G. (1980). Disability and intellectual function in multiple sclerosis. *Journal of Nervous and Mental Disease, 168,* 758-762.

Nisipeanu, P., & Korczyn, A. D. (1993). Psychological stress as risk factor for exacerbation in multiple sclerosis. *Neurology, 43*(7), 1311-1312.

Petersen, R. C., & Kokmen, E. (1989). Cognitive and psychiatric abnormalities in multiple sclerosis. *Mayo Clinic Proceedings, 64*(6), 657-663.

Pine, D. S., Douglas, C. J., Charles, E., Davies, M., & Kahn, D. (1995). Patients with multiple sclerosis presenting to psychiatric hospitals. *Journal of Clinical Psychiatry, 56*(7), 297-308.

Ron, M. A., & Logsdail, S. J. (1989). Psychiatric morbidity in multiple sclerosis: A clinical and MRI study. *Psychological Medicine, 19*(4), 887-895.

Skegg, K. (1993). Multiple sclerosis presenting as pure psychiatric disorder. *Psychological Medicine, 23*(4), 909-914.

White, D. M., Catanzaro, M. L., & Kraft, G. H. (1993). An approach to the psychological aspects of multiple sclerosis: A coping guide for health care providers and families. *Journal of Neurologic Rehabilitation, 7*(2), 43-52.

Whitlock, F. A. et al. (1980). Depression as a major symptom of multiple sclerosis. *Journal of Neurology, Neurosurgery and Psychiatry, 43,* 861-865.

Mitral Valve Prolapse

Alpert, M. A., Mukerji, V., Sabeti, M., Russell, J., & Beitman, B. D. (1991). Mitral valve prolapse, panic disorder, and chest pain. *Medical Clinics of North America, 75*(5), 1119-1133.

Bowen, R. C., D'Arcy, C., & Orchard, R. (1991). The prevalence of anxiety disorders among patients with mitral valve prolapse syndrome and chest pain. *Psychosomatics, 32*(4), 400-406.

Carney, R. M., Freedland, K. E., Ludbrook, P. A., Saunders, R. D., & Jaffe, A. S. (1990). Major depression, panic disorder, and mitral valve prolapse in patients who complain of chest pain. *American Journal of Medicine, 89*(6), 757-760.

Kaplan, A. S., Goldbloom, D. S., & Woodside, D. B. (1991). Mitral valve prolapse in eating and panic disorder: A pilot study. *International Journal of Eating Disorders, 10*(5), 531-538.

Margraf, J., Ehlers, A., & Roth, W. T. (1988). Mitral valve prolapse and panic disorder: A review of their relationship. *Psychosomatic Medicine, 50,* 93-113.

Sivaramakrishnan, K., Alexander, P. J., & Saharsarnamam, N. (1994). Prevalence of panic disorder in mitral valve prolapse: A comparative study with a cardiac control group. *Acta Psychiatrica Scandinavica, 89*(1), 59-61.

Chapter 9

Systemic Lupus Erythematosus

Adams, S. G., Dammers, P. M., et al. (1994). Stress, depression, and anxiety predict average symptom severity and daily symptom fluctuation in systemic lupus erythematosus. *Journal of Behavioral Medicine, 17,* 459-477.

Bateman, D. E. (1985). Carbamazepine induced systemic lupus erythematosis. *British Medical Journal, 291,* 632-633.

De Giorgio, C. M. et al. (1991). Carbamazepine-induced antinuclear antibodies and systemic lupus erythematosis. *Epilepsia, 32,* 128-129.

Giang, D. W. (1991). Systemic lupus erythematosis and depression. *Neuropsychiatry, Neuropsychology, and Behavioral Neurology, 4,* 78-82.

Grade, M., & Zegans, L. S. (1986). Exploring systemic lupus erythematosus: Autoimmunity, self-destruction and psychoneuroimmunology. *Advances: Institute for the Advancement of Health, 3*(2), 16-45.

Hay, E. M., Black, D., Huddy, A., Creed, F., Tomenson, B., Bernstein, R. M., & Holt, P. J. (1992). Psychiatric disorder and cognitive impairment in systemic lupus erythematosus. *Arthritis and Rheumatism, 35*(4), 411-416.

Hay, E. M., Huddy, A., Black, D., Mbaya, P., Tomenson, B., Bernstein, R. M., Lennox-Holt, P. J., & Creed, F. (1994). A prospective study of psychiatric disorder and cognitive function in systemic lupus erythematosus. *Annals of the Rheumatic Diseases, 53*(5), 298-303.

Hopkinson, N. D., Bendall, P., & Powell, R. J. (1992). Screening of acute psychiatric admissions for previously undiagnosed systemic lupus erythematosus. *British Journal of Psychiatry, 161,* 107-110.

Miguel, E. C., Pereira, R. M. R., Baer, L., Gomes, R. E., de Sá, L. C., Hirsch, R., de Barros, N. G., de Navarro, J. M., & Gentil, V. (1994). Psychiatric manifestations of systemic lupus erythematosus. *Medicine, 73*(4), 224-232.

Mitchell, W. D., & Thompson, T. L. (1990). Psychiatric distress in systemic lupus erythematosus outpatients. *Psychosomatics, 31,* 293-300.

Rogers, M. P. (1983). Psychiatric aspects. In P. H. Schur (Ed.), *The clinical management of systemic lupus erythematosus* (pp. 189-210). New York: Grune & Stratton.

Wekking, E. M. (1993). Psychiatric symptoms in systemic lupus erythematosis: An update. *Psychosomatic Medicine, 55,* 219-228.

Hypoglycemia

Bondy, P. K., & Felig, P. (1974). Disorders of carbohydrate metabolism. In P. K. Bondy & I. E. Rosenberg (Eds.), *Duncan's disease of metabolism* (7th ed.). Philadelphia: W. B. Saunders.

Harp, M. J. (1990). Correlations of the physical symptoms of hypoglycemia with the psychological symptoms of anxiety and depression. *Journal of Orthomolecular Medicine, 5*(1), 8-10.

Klonoff, E. A., & Biglan, A. (1987). "Hypoglycemic" anxiety: The role of reinforcement in psychophysiological disorders. *Behavior Modification, 11,* 102-113.

Young-Hyman, D., & Mersey, H. (1994). Evaluation of the unexplained symptoms of hypoglycemia. *Maryland Medical Journal, 43*(6), 523-526.

Wilson's Disease

Dening, T. R., & Berrios, G. E. (1990). Wilson's disease: A longitudinal study of psychiatric symptoms. *Biological Psychiatry, 28*(3), 255-265.

Jackson, G. H., Meyer, A., & Lippmann, S. (1994). Wilson's disease: Psychiatric manifestations may be the clinical presentation. *Postgraduate Medicine, 95*(8), 135-138.

Marsden, C. D. (1987). Wilson's disease. *Quarterly Journal of Medicine, 65,* 959-966.

Walker, S. (1969). The psychiatric presentation of Wilson's disease (hepatolenticular degeneration) with an etiologic explanation. *Behavioral Neuropsychiatry, 1,* 38-43.

Walshe, J. M. (1988). Diagnosis and treatment of presymptomatic Wilson's disease. *Lancet, 2,* 435-437.

Cancer of the Pancreas

Fras, I., Litin, E. M., & Bartholamew, L. G. (1968). Mental symptoms as an aid in the early diagnosis of carcinoma of the pancreas. *Gastroenterology,* 191-198.

Kelsen, D. P., Portenoy, R. K., Thaler, W. T., Niedzwiecki, D., Passik, S. D., Tao, Y., Banks., Brennan, M. F., & Foley, K. M. (1995). Pain and depression in patients with newly diagnosed pancreas cancer. *Journal of Clinical Oncology, 13*(3), 748-755.

Knowlessar, O. D. (1975). Diseases of the pancreas. In P. B. Beeson & W. McDermott (Eds.), *Textbook of medicine* (14th ed., p. 1250). Philadelphia: W. B. Saunders.

Schuster, M. M., & Iber, F. L. (1965). Psychosis with pancreatitis. *Archives of Internal Medicine,* 228-233.

Pheochromocytoma

Benowitz, N. L. (1990). Phaeochromocytoma. *Advances in Internal Medicine, 35,* 195-219.

Fogarty, J., Engel, C. C., & Russo, J. (1994). Hypertension and phaeochromocytoma testing: The association with anxiety disorders. *Archives of Family Medicine, 3*(1), 55-60.

Lambert, M. T. (1992). Phaeochromocytoma presenting as exacerbation of post-traumatic stress Disorder symptomology. *International Journal of Psychiatry in Medicine, 22*(3), 265-268.

Starkman, M. N., Cameron, O. G., Nesse, R. M., & Zelnik, T. (1990). Peripheral catecholamine levels and the symptoms of anxiety: Studies in patients with and without phaeochromocytoma. *Psychosomatic Medicine, 52*(2), 129-142.

Index

Paraphilias, temporal lobe epilepsy and, 115
Parathyroid glands, 5, 6
    definition of, 127
    disorders of, 23-24
    See also Hypoparathyroidism;
        Hypocalcemia
Parkinson's disease, 39-40
Partial (focal) seizures, simple, 31, 43, 45,
        124
    adversive, 46
    auditory sensory, 46
    definition of, 127
    focal motor, 45-46, 124
    misdiagnosis of, 46-51
    postural, 46, 127
    somatic sensory, 46
    vertiginous, 46
    visual sensory, 46
    with elementary motor symptoms, 45-46
    with elementary sensory symptoms, 46
Peripheral neuropathy, definition of, 127
Personality disorders:
    hyperparathyroidism/hypercalcemia and,
        115
    hypopituitarism and, 115
    multiple sclerosis and, 115
    ruling out physical causes of, 119
    temporal lobe epilepsy and, 115
Petit mal seizures:
    absence attacks during, 43-44
    automatism during, 44
    definition of, 127
    in children, 43
    length of, 43
    Lennox-Gastaut syndrome and, 44
Pheochromocytoma, 92
    definition of, 127
Pituitary gland, 5-6
    definition of, 127
    disorders, 6, 22-23
    See also Hypopituitarism
Polefrone, J., 110
Polyglandular insufficiency syndromes, 8
    definition of, 127
Popkin, M. K., xxi
Poriomania, 66
    definition of, 127
Posterolateral sclerosis, 89
    conversion disorder and, 115
    definition of, 127
    generalized anxiety disorder and, 114
Postictal seizure stage, 30, 44, 54

complex automatisms during, 61
hypersexuality during, 62
length of, 61
simple automatisms during, 61
violence during, 62
Price, R. H., xxiii
Primary seizure disorders, 30
    causes of, 30
Primictal seizure stage, 30, 54, 55
    complex auditory musical hallucinations
        during, 56-57, 59
    complex auditory verbal hallucinations
        during, 57-59
    complex visual illusions during, 60
    definition of, 127
    déjà vu during, 60
    depersonalization during, 60
    derealization during, 60
    elementary auditory hallucinations during,
        56
    elementary auditory illusions during, 56
    elementary visual illusions during, 59-60
    gustatory hallucinations during, 60
    jamais vu during, 60
    olfactory hallucinations during, 60
    paliacousia type of verbal hallucinations
        during, 58-59
Prodromal seizure stage, 30
    definition of, 127
    length of, 54-55
    PMS and, 55
    symptoms, 55
Psychiatric disorders:
    and possible physical disorders, 114-115
Psychomotor epilepsy, definition of, 127
Pugliesi, K., xxvii

Radziunas, E., 89
Regier, D. A., xxvii
Reifman, A., xxvii
Repetti, R. L., xxvii
Rickel, A. U., xxii
Rittenhouse, Joan, xxi
Robins, L. N., xxvii
Role conflict, xxiii
Role overload, xxiii
Rorschach, xv
Russo, N. F., xxii, xxiii, xxvii

Sacks, O., 38

About the Authors

Elizabeth A. Klonoff, a clinical and health psychologist, received her PhD in clinical psychology from the University of Oregon in 1977. She was Director of the Behavioral Medicine Clinic at University Hospitals of Cleveland, Case Western Reserve University Medical School (1979-1988), and is currently Professor of Psychology and Executive Director of the Behavioral Health Institute at California State University-San Bernardino. In addition to teaching and acting as director of the Institute, she conducts numerous, grant-supported research projects on sexism, racism, and physical and mental health. She has published widely on culture and gender diversity in clinical psychology, behavioral medicine, and preventive medicine. Her most recent books include *African-American Acculturation: Deconstructing Race and Reviving Culture* (1996, Sage) and *Sexist Discrimination in Women's Lives* (1997, Sage, forthcoming), both with Hope Landrine.

Hope Landrine received her PhD in clinical psychology from the University of Rhode Island (1983), completed postdoctoral training in social psychology at Stanford University (1984-1986), and received additional training in preventive medicine in the Department of Preventive Medicine, University of Southern California Medical School (1992-1993). She is currently a Research Scientist at the Public Health Foundation (of Los Angeles County) where she conducts full-time, grant-supported research and preventive interventions on the health of women, girls, and ethnic minorities. She has published widely on culture and gender diversity in preventive medicine and in clinical and health psychology. Her other books include *The Politics of Madness* (1992), *Bringing Cultural Diversity to Feminist Psychology* (1995), and (with Elizabeth Klonoff) *African-American Acculturation: Deconstructing Race and Reviving Culture* (1996, Sage) and *Sexist Discrimination in Women's Lives* (1997, Sage, forthcoming).